OPERATOR SYNDROME

OPERATOR SYNDROME

CHRIS FRUEH, PhD

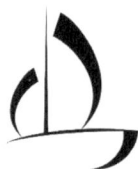

Ballast Books, LLC
www.ballastbooks.com

ISBN: 978-1-962202-07-7

Printed in Hong Kong

Published by Ballast Books
www.ballastbooks.com

For more information, bulk orders, appearances, or speaking requests, please email: info@ballastbooks.com

DEDICATION

For Claude E. Brocklebank and Mrs. John R. Beane

SPECIAL THANKS TO:

All the men and women who have served within the special operations community of democratic nations; all the men and women from the SOF community who have talked with me over the years; all those who spoke on the record and are quoted within this book; Operator Syndrome Foundation (David and Jana Rutherford, Dan Cerillo); SEAL Future Foundation (Johnny Wilson, Paul Polakowski, Ty Bathurst, Paul Thoma, Bradford Peters), the SFF Health team (Joey Fio, Justin Hoagland, David Bruchu), and the SFF Health Board of Advisors (Richard Auchus, Carol Bender, Denise Bottiglieri, Jenn Byrne, Rebecca Ivory, Karen Kelly, Robert Koffman, Kevin Lacz, Gabrielle Lyon, Sean Mulvaney, Kirk Parsley); Military Special Operations Family Collaborative (KaLea Lehman, Lindsey Snook); The Mission Within (Martin Polanco, Robert Ryan); Heroic Hearts (Jesse Gould); VETS, Inc. (Marcus and Amber Capone); Boulder Crest Foundation (Ken Falke, Josh Goldberg); my first two SOF health mentors, Joe Bonvie and George Steffian; SOF or SOF-adjacent colleagues who profoundly influenced my understanding, including Geoff Dardia, Bryan Stepanenko, and Gary Hoyt; my collaborators on the 2020 paper published in *The International Journal of Psychiatry in Medicine* (Alok Madan, J. Christopher Fowler, Sasha Stomberg, Major Bradshaw, Karen Kelly, Benjamin Weinstein, Morgan Luttrell, Summer G. Danner, Deborah C. Beidel); Jadie Miller and Brad Wylie of PYROC Technologies; Isabella Zingray, project manager; Jeff Smith, U.S. military historian; Andy Symonds, my editor and publisher at Ballast Books; Sonia Land, my fiction literary agent (London); Robert and Char Ekoniak; Tyler Black; and my dear wife, Karen L. Pellegrin.

"I feel uniquely made with no one to understand the war still going on inside my head and heart."
—**Brandon Cruz**, former U.S. Navy SEAL

"Operator Syndrome. Maybe you do not like or understand the term. Maybe you feel it singles out one group for special attention. I do not see it this way, but that is fine. I see it as a starting point to bring the matter to the table for discussion. The syndrome described in this book is a real issue for many soldiers post-military service. Why not engage, debate, learn, and educate ourselves, in order to hopefully help others?"
—**Jeff White**, U.S. Army Sergeant Major, former Special Missions Unit Operator

TABLE OF CONTENTS

FOREWORD

To My Operator Brothers, the season of death is again upon us. And once again, it is incumbent on us to thwart its grasp.

For more than twenty years, my friends, family, and brothers have shown that the country's call would not go unheard. The Global War on Terror delivered to our great nation a call to arms, a call to fight an ideological war against an amorphous, concealed, and antipathetic enemy driven by the hatred of our way of life. Each of you understands intimately how our war cost the lifeblood of so many honorable men. The magnitude of their deeds has brilliantly memorialized their sacrifices. Our country once portrayed us as their saviors, reliant on our devotion to serve each other, as well as the oath that governs our very existence. However, we and our families are now drowning in the uneven tides of a nation seemingly oblivious to our sacrifices, and the indifferent leaders of the same government that sent us to fight in faraway lands. The abrupt and disastrous abandonment of Afghanistan further underscores this callous disregard for our sacrifices and those of our local allies in-country.

For these reasons, as well as the recognition of my own personal struggles, I believe it is up to us—those who seek to lighten the burden of our anguish—to make sure that we shall not fall into the proverbial abyss of history's forgotten soldiers. It is with great pride that I scribe this letter for Chris Frueh, a true champion of our well-being. The honor imbued within his words is unconditional, and the gratitude he feels toward all of us is infinite. The time has come to invest our lives, once again, beyond the scope of our committed oath, and to push forth unto the breach, beyond which there are answers to our immense struggles and, with God's great blessings, the help our fellow warriors need to find peace amidst the shattering complexities of Operator Syndrome.

Written in the spirit of our devotion to serving others, this book sets forth to provide the committed assistance and understanding to the special operators themselves—we who so desperately need and want it. We shall bring forth the totality of our greatest attributes, lessons learned, and genuine servitude toward our brothers-in-arms, in order to deliver each man back to the path of his salvation. We are forever on the precipice of war, yet without our unwavering resolve to heal those who have already fought, the next generation will lose faith in the reciprocation promised in exchange for their resolve. We cannot let that happen.

Thank you, Chris, for your unquestionable love of our nation— and thanks to all the men who chose to fight the great evils in our midst. We have your back, as you have ours. Godspeed.

And to those Americans who truly want to know: Every American who loves this great nation should commit themselves, at the very least, to understanding the monumental sacrifices made by our Special Operations Forces (SOF) members. For more than twenty years, the SOF community has unrelentingly answered the call in the Global War on Terror. These elite warfighters have borne the primary burden of waging war across multiple continents and countless nations. Year after year, battle after battle, sacrifice after sacrifice, they provided the human resources our nation needed to hunt the enemy on their own lands. The price they are paying for the government's ambition is devastating.

I am a former operator who suffers from Operator Syndrome. This book fully explains and describes the hell so many of our nation's most elite warfighters are living with daily. As you read, think about the life you are living, the beauty of your freedom and family, and the sanctity of your security. You enjoy these God-given rights because of the people who are willing to wage war for you and on your family's behalf. Now it is time for you to sacrifice for them. This sacrifice begins with the time you commit to understanding the magnitude of their challenges. God willing, once you realize the harrowing nature of their irreversible exposures, you will seek and find ways to serve them, as they have served you.

Thank you and God bless you.

Most Sincerely,
David Rutherford
former U.S. Navy SEAL, CIA contractor,
cofounder of the Operator Syndrome Foundation

INTRODUCTION

I n the fall of 1898, Mrs. John R. Beane traveled up to Montauk Point, Long Island. She was almost certainly traveling in a horse-drawn carriage, and she was probably accompanied by a butler and other retinue.

The Spanish-American War had just ended, and American soldiers were coming home. Camp Wikoff[1] had been established that August as an isolation camp to hold the men returning from Cuba and Puerto Rico, many of whom were sick with yellow fever, malaria, dysentery, and other communicable tropical diseases.

Lasting only two months that year, the war in the Cuban theater had been brief (June 10 to August 7), and U.S. combat casualties had been relatively light (fewer than four hundred killed and 1,500 wounded). However, over two thousand U.S. soldiers had died of disease while in theater, and tens of thousands of returning soldiers were gravely ill with highly infectious mosquito-borne diseases.

Camp Wikoff had been established just weeks before returning troops began to arrive, and the camp had never been properly completed. It was overwhelmed by the large number of sick and malnourished troops; at one point the camp

---

1   Camp Wikoff was named after Colonel Charles A. Wikoff, 22nd U.S. Infantry, who was killed July 1, 1898, in an assault on the San Juan Heights.

held over twenty thousand soldiers. Conditions at the camp, with its rows of rudimentary tents, were so poor that President William McKinley felt compelled to visit and see for himself.

Mrs. Beane traveled up from her home in New York City, possibly as part of a larger civilian grassroots effort. When she reached the overflowing camp, she identified several men who were very ill—strangers to her—and brought them home with her. There she nursed them for weeks, and then, when they were ready and healthy enough to travel, she helped them get home. Not only was this act extremely generous, her treatment also risked infection spreading to her and her own family.

One of the soldiers, Claude Emmett Brocklebank, spent six weeks under Mrs. Beane's care at her home. At age seventeen, he had left either an orphanage or a foster care home, lied about his age, volunteered with the U.S. Army, been deployed to Cuba in Company F's 34th Michigan Volunteers, and fought at the Battle of San Juan and Kettle Hills. Yet it was after his combat experience that Claude faced the greatest threat. For the rest of his life, he would quite reasonably believe that it was Mrs. Beane who had saved his life.

Claude had already served his country, and now so had she.

It was an era preceding the federal Department of Veterans Affairs. At that time, there was little more than a patchwork of state-run domiciliary-care veterans homes. Fortunately for the soldiers who had deployed to Cuba, the civilian-military divide then was a small fraction of what it has since become in the U.S.

For more than 250 years, it was accepted that civilians played an important role in caring for the men who had fought on their behalf. This tradition traces back to 1636, when the Pilgrims of Plymouth Colony passed a law requiring the people of the colony to care for soldiers injured or disabled in the war with the Pequot Indians. Many civilians rightly considered it their responsibility to help care for the nation's warriors. Mrs. John R. Beane was part of that long tradition.

Claude Brocklebank was my great-grandfather. He lived to be almost one hundred years old, and I got to know him during my childhood before he died when I was fourteen. Some of what I know about him has been passed down through family lore, but much of it I heard directly from him.

He described to me the austere conditions in Cuba. I learned that he and his unit took much of the fire from the Spanish troops above them on Kettle and San Juan Hills, while Teddy Roosevelt and his "Rough Riders" ran up the back of the hills and captured the defensive positions. It bothered him that Roosevelt and his boys got most of the credit and glory for the victory, while the units at the front base of the hills had taken most of the U.S. casualties. My great-grandfather's personal accounts of the war and his return home have inspired me ever since.

———

Before I continue, I should offer a brief word on my background and what led me to write this book: I was born in 1963 and grew up in the shadow of the Vietnam War. My father was a U.S. Air Force physician and Vietnam veteran. As a family, we attended Quaker meetings throughout much of the 1970s, which meant I was raised with a strong "conscientious objector" perspective toward war.

With a desire to serve the veteran community, I earned a doctorate in clinical psychology in 1992. Over the past thirty years, I've worked as a therapist at a Veterans Affairs hospital's PTSD clinic, held tenured professorships at two medical schools and one state university, applied for and received millions of dollars in federal grants, directed large research programs, and published over three hundred scientific papers, including a graduate textbook on psychopathology.

Some years ago, a friend of mine who had recently transitioned out of the Navy confided in me. His career included about fifteen years as a Navy SEAL, including time with the Naval Special Warfare Development Group (DEVGRU), or SEAL Team Six, participating in a number of their mission sets. When he said to me, "I don't feel like myself anymore," I naively thought that I, a so-called PTSD "expert," could help him—*except that he did not have PTSD.*

Over the course of many conversations, various medical tests, and a lot of trial and error, it emerged that his difficulties stemmed from physiological pathologies more than psychopathologies.

This realization begged multiple questions:

Why would an elite warfighter in his late thirties have low testosterone—and what else was going on in his body?

If our reliance on the PTSD diagnosis is misguided, should we instead use an approach that considers all of the body's physiological systems?

In the years since that first conversation, I have talked and worked with hundreds of military special operators, often on a regular basis over the course of years, and I have developed many close relationships in the community. In 2020, several of my colleagues and I published a medical journal paper that attempted to describe and make sense of the interrelated constellation of medical conditions, injuries, impairments, and social difficulties we had seen. We gave this whole systems framework a name that we and many others had already been informally using for years: Operator Syndrome.

This book is for the Special Operations Forces (SOF) community—the operators and their spouses—so that they may better understand the nature of their difficulties, as well as the many powerful therapies that can help alleviate suffering and return them to a higher level of health and elite performance. Operators are a community of highly intelligent problem solvers, and I have no doubt they will be able to make good use of this information and continue to lead in the search for solutions.

I also hope that readers outside the SOF community will develop a greater appreciation of the incredible sacrifices that a very small group of elite warfighters and their families have made on our collective behalf.

PART ONE

THE SYNDROME

CHAPTER 1

OPERATOR SYNDROME

"Every time I see a new primary doctor, VA or civilian, they are completely overwhelmed by the sheer number and severity of the different medical issues I have. Nobody knows how to treat me. I'm completely different from any other patient they've had.

"For over ten years I struggled to understand why I am the way I am, and to know what was really wrong with me. Then I came across an article on Operator Syndrome and was like, 'Holy shit, I'm normal!' I went from feeling totally alone to being part of the tribe again.

"It's hard to quantify the change I have experienced in the last year to simply understanding that I wasn't just 'fucked up.' Knowing I wasn't alone in that I was dealing with some very heavy things, and knowing that there was a community forming to tackle them together, gave me hope. I've been able to access care that isn't widely known, or even 'authorized' yet for certain conditions."

—**Clay Jensen**, U.S. Army Master Sergeant (Ret.), Special Operations Team-Alpha (SOT-A), 7th Special Forces Group, Other Government Agency (CIA) contractor, with seven deployments to combat zones from 2001 to 2008

"No one warned us about this. As a SEAL wife, I knew that I could lose him or that he could come back wounded or without limbs. These were the hard realities I actually prepared for. But no one ever told us that they would come back from war, looking perfectly fine, and be so completely changed. That our future would be so drastically altered by silent injuries. It makes recovery that much harder because no one thinks anything is wrong, the Operators included."

—**Tania Beaudoin**, licensed clinical social worker, U.S. Navy SEAL spouse

*"When I teach current and prior operators about Operator Syndrome, I see lightbulb moments in the room, which is usually followed by an intense sense of relief. So many of them have been told over and over again that there is **nothing wrong** with them—that their MRI was normal, or their T-levels were normal (according to the branch's standard), and that it must be PTSD or some other mental health 'issue.'"*

—**Dr. Jennifer Byrne**, U.S. Air Force veteran, Special Operations spouse

"When educating operators on Operator Syndrome, the most common response is: 'How did you know?' This response is usually expressed with a tone of relief and a subtle smile. For the operator, it marks a moment of validation and a glimmer of hope: 'Maybe I'm not alone.' Understanding that their brain is injured and they aren't broken illuminates a light at the end of the tunnel."

—**Hoagie**, Special Operator (Ret.)

Imagine a male medical patient in his late thirties who describes the following symptoms to his doctor: low mood, insomnia, irritability, low motivation, low energy, and poor concentration. The patient's expression is flat, and his face looks weary. His shoulders are slumped a little, and he stares at the floor a lot. During the clinical interview, he acknowledges that he has been drinking heavily for the past few months and arguing more with his girlfriend. He doesn't understand what is wrong with him. He's never been like this before.

In most modern medical settings, this patient is virtually guaranteed to receive a diagnosis of major depressive disorder and probably at least one or two other psychiatric disorders. If he's a service member or veteran, he's also likely to be diagnosed with PTSD. Prescriptions will quickly follow. Over a short period of time, the patient is likely to find himself with a daily regimen of at least two antidepressant medications (Prozac? Wellbutrin? Effexor?), sleeping pills (Ambien? Prazosin?), and possibly a mood stabilizer (Lamotrigine?), a benzodiazepine (Xanax?), or both. Many veterans report being prescribed over twenty different medications at a time by VA clinicians.

The doctor will also probably refer the patient for psychotherapy, typically with a social worker or masters-level mental health counselor. The patient will then likely sit on a waiting list for up to three or four months—or even more. When finally seen, his therapist will be well-intentioned, supportive, thoughtful, even kind. They will encourage the patient to adopt a psychological perspective toward his suffering. *It's all in your head*, they might suggest. The therapist will likely coax the patient to talk at length about his childhood and adult experiences. The focus will be on adverse, stressful, or traumatic experiences, past and current. The therapist will also put an emphasis on relationships and negative emotions, questioning at every session about suicidal thoughts and the presence of firearms in the patient's home.

But what if the root cause of this patient's torturous symptoms is a severe pathophysiological dysfunction—at the molecular and cellular level—which can be identified with a simple blood test? For example, what if he has an endocrine disorder—specifically hypogonadism? Very low testosterone could cause all of the symptoms he described, but virtually no practitioner in the mental health field routinely checks for hormonal dysregulation. This almost never happens! Neither Veterans Affairs (VA) nor the Department of Defense (DOD) include hormone blood lab panels as part of their standard operating procedures.

Obviously, being treated for depression while you have a missed diagnosis of hypogonadism almost certainly means you are being treated for the wrong illness. Important insights might still emerge from therapeutic conversations. Psychiatric medications may help a little, although it is also quite likely that prescribing psychiatric medications for a pathophysiological dysfunction will cause more problems than it solves.

What would we think of a baseball batting coach attempting to help hitters by focusing primarily on their childhood, adverse life experiences, emotions, and relationship history—all while ignoring the physical aspects of human performance? We would think that coach is unlikely to be of much use to individual players or to the rest of the team.

———————

Over the past thirty years, I've been a faculty member at several large, multidisciplinary academic medical school psychiatry departments, and not one of them had an endocrinologist. The faculty included psychiatrists, psychologists, nurses, social workers, statisticians, sociologists, and even geneticists—but no endocrinologists.

More broadly, the entire mental health field seems to have carved itself apart from the rest of biology and medicine. Rather than hear a patient's "psychological" symptoms as certain evidence of "psychopathology," perhaps it is time to understand that many psychological or social difficulties are second- and third-order effects of pathology elsewhere in the body?

I and many others believe that we must take a whole systems approach. This obviously includes the nervous system, but it should also not overlook the endocrine, musculoskeletal, perceptual, pulmonary, digestive, and cardiac systems, as well as others. Beyond the body, there are family, community, and occupational systems, and for the SOF community specifically, there are systems to consider within military units, transition services, Veteran Affairs, and other organizations—again, a truly whole systems approach

In our 2020 medical journal article, several of us proposed a framework to better understand and address the complex and unique injuries sustained during a typical career in military special operations:

> *Operator Syndrome* may be understood as the natural consequences of an extraordinarily high allostatic load; the accumulation of physiological, neural, and neuroendocrine responses resulting from the prolonged chronic stress; and physical demands of a career with the military special forces.[2]

---

2   Christopher Frueh, et al, "'Operator Syndrome': A unique constellation of medical and behavioral healthcare needs of military special operations forces," *The International Journal of Psychiatry in Medicine* 55, no. 4 (2020): 281–295.

None of this is to say that mental health concerns are not relevant to operators; they most certainly are, and in a variety of ways. But the heavy emphasis we have placed on psychiatric disorders, particularly in the context of a SOF suicide epidemic, is misguided. We've placed PTSD—and, to a lesser extent, other psychiatric disorders—in the foreground, while allowing other chronic medical problems to drift into the background, where they often go ignored and forgotten.

I believe it is time we switch this foregrounded emphasis on psychiatric illness with the overlooked background of physiological injuries, chronic medical problems, and social challenges. Against traditional diagnoses and treatments, my opinion may seem counterintuitive, but I believe that an exclusive focus on *psychiatric disorders* fails to address many of the root causes of mounting SOF suicides.

––––––––––

The military special operations community is unlike any other. They have unique selection and training, undergo unique mission sets, sustain unique injuries, and require unique solutions. They are American military heroes who have spent more than twenty years fighting the Global War on Terror (GWOT) all over the world. Their individual and collective accomplishments are legendary—as they deserve to be. Memoirs and histories have been written about them. Movies and television shows have been made celebrating their deeds.

The general public typically regards them as elite, brave, thrilling, sexy. They are held in awe by many. People admire them and want to be associated with them, not unlike the way rock stars and athletes are idolized. This is completely understandable!

At the same time, however, relatively few of us understand the massive "dose" of allostatic load they have shouldered for our benefit as Americans. Few understand the depth, complexity, and intensity, both physical and mental, of their sacrifices, involving brain, body, and soul. Most people cannot imagine it.

Moreover, resentments have developed in some quarters. Some believe the SOF have been treated as "special" for long enough, and that going forward, they should receive the exact same medical services as other soldiers and veterans. One prominent neurologist told me it would be a "social injustice" to provide them with specialty medical care designed to target their unique injuries. Other critics go so far as to say we should be wary of their "toxic masculinity" and possible war crimes.

What Is a Military Special Operator and Why Are They Unique?

Military special operators are elite warriors, making up less than 1 percent of the U.S. Armed Forces. A similar ratio is found among the militaries of other NATO countries. Their selection and training are incredibly demanding and rigorous. For most SOF units, less than 10 percent of those who attempt selection courses are able to pass. Contrary to the common stereotype of a "knuckle dragger," operators are not only physically and mentally tough, but also highly intelligent and creative problem solvers.

In the U.S., special operations are organized under Special Operations Command (SOCOM) and its subordinate command, Joint Special Operations Command (JSOC). Approximately seventy thousand men and women make up this force, including operators, intelligence officers, aviators, civil affairs personnel, psychological operations specialists, highly skilled technical enablers, explosive ordinance disposal (EODs) technicians, and officers. Almost 100 percent of operators are male, but there are females throughout SOCOM and the intelligence community. There are even several female Army Rangers.

Each branch of the U.S. military has their own special operations units. These include, but are not limited to, the following:

- **Army:** The 75th Ranger Regiment, Special Forces (a.k.a. Green Berets), Special Operations Aviation Regiment (SOAR; a.k.a. Night Stalkers)
- **Air Force:** Pararescue (a.k.a. PJs), Combat Control, Special Reconnaissance, Tactical Air Control Party
- **Marine Corps:** Marine Corps Forces Special Operations Command (MARSOC; a.k.a. Marine Raiders)
- **Navy:** SEALs, Special Warfare Combatant-Craft (SWCC), Explosive and Ordinance Disposal (EOD)
- **Coast Guard:** Deployable Operations Group

Under JSOC, most of the branches have at least a single Tier One unit, with unique selection processes and special mission sets. Examples include Navy's DEVGRU (a.k.a. SEAL Team Six), the Army's 1st Special Forces Operational Detachment-Delta (a.k.a. Delta Force), and the Air Force's 24th Special Tactics Squadron (24th STS).

Most of the U.S. intelligence agencies (e.g., Central Intelligence Agency, Defense Intelligence Agency) and law enforcement agencies (e.g., Drug Enforcement Agency) also have paramilitary operators, cryptographers, and intelligence officers integrated within JSOC units and operations.

Other units and roles within the western defense community have similarities to the formally recognized special operations elements. Marine infantry units, private defense contractors, combat aviators, combat divers, snipers, EOD, paratroopers, and others may sustain similar injuries as those in special operations. Within SOCOM, there are also civil affairs, psyops, and other important roles that face similar risks.

Cultural Support Teams comprised of female combatants are an especially under-recognized and underserved group. They deployed alongside special operations units in Afghanistan and Iraq, with the primary responsibility of engaging local females in operational areas, including on targets. They embedded and worked with SOF units, sharing in the dangers, exposures, and downstream injuries.

Many private defense contractors (often former U.S. military operators) functioned like operators in their contract work. There are several important things most people don't know about defense contractors: Not all of them are operators—some are local interpreters (e.g., Iraqi or Afghani nationals), mechanics, logistics and operations management, among other roles. Many of them serve between five and fifteen years, or even more, within a war zone. Finally, because of their status outside of the military, the VA system does not recognize them, so these contractors have no visibility, public support, societal recognition, or benefits. Some estimates indicate that about half of those who supported the U.S. military efforts in Afghanistan and Iraq were private defense contractors. *This means there are a lot of them, and yet they remain invisible to most Americans.*

There are many published histories and memoirs that provide a far better account of the experience of military special operators than I possibly can. There are dozens of excellent books written about SOF selection (including the Army's Q Course or the Navy's BUDS), training, tactics, weapons and technology, deployments, missions, and individual careers. I won't try to summarize or replicate this body of literature. But I will provide a short overview of the career experiences and features that contribute to the unique constellation of injuries commonly incurred in the course of a career in special operations.

Blast Exposures

Most operators receive intensive training in demolitions and breaching, spending months at a time in close proximity to explosions and the overpressure caused by blast waves. They also receive extensive training in multiple weapons systems (e.g., Carl Gustaf rifles that fire rockets) that involve additional massive blast exposures. Even firing a rifle or a handgun involves a micro-blast exposure, and these add up over the course of tens of thousands of rounds fired. These blast exposures are cumulative, much in the same way that concussions and impact force blows are to the head. It has been estimated that greater than 85 percent of operators sustain a traumatic brain injury from training alone—before they are ever even deployed to an operational theater. The cumulative "dose" of blast wave exposure over the course of an operator's career is usually several orders of magnitude greater than it is for soldiers in conventional forces.

High Operational Tempo and Chronic Stress

The GWOT has largely been a war fought by special operations forces, with deployed conventional forces playing an important support role. It has been overlooked and downplayed, so I'll say the quiet part out loud: Estimates suggest that SOF have been responsible for 95 percent of the combat over the past twenty plus years. Many operators have upwards of twelve or more deployments, typically of three to nine months' duration, with hundreds of missions. Some have over a thousand missions during their career. These deployments typically involved going out on one or more missions a night for weeks or months at a time. Moreover, when not deployed, operators constantly undergo rigorous and demanding training evolutions.

Violence of Action

Few people understand the extreme danger and violence SOF deployments and missions entail. It's not uncommon for operators to be shot at and to kill enemy combatants or insurgents on a frequent, even nightly, basis while deployed. Many operators have killed literally hundreds of people in close quarters combat during their career. Special operations have also taken the brunt of the casualties during the GWOT. Most operators and their families have lost dozens of comrades and attended numerous military funerals. Some still carry the phone numbers of their dead in their mobile phones.

Training

The skills and training required to conduct complex, stealthy missions are demanding and dangerous. Operators receive extensive training in rucking, diving, parachute jumping, rappelling, and tactical combat driving. They learn how to fight, maneuver, and survive in the most austere environments. Most receive training in survival, evasion, resistance, and escape during the SERE program. The risk of injury and death, even during training, is significant.

Orthopedic Injuries

Obviously, the physical wear and tear over time, as well as acute injury risk, is massive. It is not uncommon for an operator to have multiple orthopedic surgeries over the course of their career, and most live with chronic pain in their neck, shoulders, elbows, wrists, back, hips, knees, and ankles. Virtually every joint in their body may be injured by the end of their service.

Toxic Exposures

The risk of burn-pit exposures faced by all soldiers in the military has received quite a bit of attention in recent years. For SOF, the list of other potentially toxic exposures is additionally very high. This includes chronic exposure to many different heavy metals, environmental toxins and gases, smoke, chemicals in uniform materials, biological and radiological elements, and poor-quality air, food, and water. Several operators I know have independently described remote locations with exposed "neon green ponds," once used by prior armies (e.g., from the Soviet era) or more recent insurgents. One operator was diagnosed with type 1 diabetes several years after his deployment, which is unusual, and he wondered if it was connected to toxic exposures in the area.

Career Length and Time Away from Home

While most soldiers in conventional military forces complete enlistments of four years, while a much smaller percentage complete twenty-year careers, a high percentage of operators are in for the long haul—*at least* twenty years—unless they are too injured to continue. The average age of a Tier One operator is typically mid to late thirties. Moreover, with deployments and off-site training evolutions, operators can expect to be far away from home throughout most of their career, commonly around nine months out of every year. Many operators estimate they have missed 80 percent of family birthdays, holidays, and milestones.

Compartmentalizing Pain: The "Never Quit" Culture

The SOF community are the people who "mount up and ride to the sound of the guns." No soldier in any branch of the U.S. military can be ordered to serve in SOF. Operators are entirely volunteer. They self-select for the job, the mission, and the life. Selection processes are designed to push even the toughest applicants to quit and return to conventional forces. Pain comes with the job, and operators effectively compartmentalize that pain. They stoically push through and ignore the pain, and as a consequence, most of their non-acute injuries are left untreated for years, sometimes until the very end of a career. Because of the popular perception of their invincibility, as a society, we rarely offer a hand when they need help. This means injuries and impairments accrue untended as the years of training evolutions, deployments, and missions add up.

Operators live by the principle to "never quit," to "never give up," and to "never be out of the fight." Every major branch and unit have their ethos, slogans, emblems, and patches. I won't detail them here, because there are so many of them, but a common feature is a focus on dedication to one's brothers-in-arms. The late Navy SEAL Bradley S. Cavner neatly summarized the commitment to the SOF brotherhood with the following toast:

> To those before us, to those amongst us, to those we'll see on the other side. Lord, let me not prove unworthy of my brothers.

Allostatic Load—"Whole Systems" Approach

The phrase "allostatic load" refers to a theoretical construct representing the cumulative burden of chronic physical and psychological stressors. A career in SOF clearly involves regular exposure to chronic stress, violence and danger, and a wide range of physiological injuries, including traumatic brain injuries. The accumulation of these physiological, physical, psychological, and neuroendocrine injuries (i.e., high allostatic load) can lead to profound physiological changes upon the individual. I believe it leads to a profession-specific constellation of interrelated medical, social, and psychological conditions. A whole systems framework can help us better understand and address the complex medical and behavioral healthcare needs of operators.

Operator Syndrome: A Brief Overview

Operator Syndrome is a unique constellation of interrelated medical, psychological, and social conditions commonly found in military special operators. It includes traumatic brain injury, endocrine dysfunction, sleep disturbance and sleep disorders, chronic pain and headaches, depression, anxiety, anger, hypervigilance, PTSD, substance abuse, perceptual systems impairments, cognitive impairments, marital and family concerns, intimacy concerns, military-civilian transition concerns, existential concerns, and the potential effects of toxic exposures. (The original medical paper on Operator Syndrome can be found online with a quick key word search, and it is a quick and easy read—really!)

Operator Syndrome is a whole systems framework that can be used both to optimize performance and to address the complex downstream injuries of a career in military special operations. While each medical domain can be evaluated *individually* by medical specialists, I believe there is value in having a short and practical instrument to rate these conditions as a *whole*—as a *syndrome*. For this reason, we developed the Operator Syndrome Scale. This public-domain instrument may be used by operators and spouses to do the following:

1. Learn about Operator Syndrome.
2. Help you reach a better understanding of your health, wellness, and functioning.
3. Facilitate conversations with yourself and your partner.
4. Initiate and guide conversations with your primary care provider and other medical specialists.

A Few Thoughts on PTSD

I'm sure most of you are familiar with PTSD, a very common psychiatric disorder among military veterans. It is one of the go-to diagnoses for the VA healthcare system. So, what is it exactly? Post-traumatic stress disorder (PTSD) is a psychiatric illness caused by exposure to "traumatic" experiences. The simplest way to describe PTSD is that it is a combination of depression and anxiety, plus symptoms of trauma-specific fear reactivity.

"Fear reactivity" includes intrusive and distressing memories about the trauma, nightmares, "flashbacks," anxiety at reminders of the trauma, and avoidance of external reminders of the trauma. The good news for sufferers is that a large body of research literature shows that PTSD is a highly treatable disorder with behavioral therapies, at least in civilian and non-VA veteran populations.

Operator Syndrome Scale
Short Form

Operator's Name: _____   **Date:** _____

Instructions: Below is a list of difficulties that some people who served in military special operations experience. Please use the totality of information available to you, including medical records and tests that you are aware of, as well as your own perspective to make ratings.

		Unable to Rate	None	Mild	Moder-ate	Severe
1	Traumatic Brain Injury		0	1	2	3
2	Sleep Disturbance		0	1	2	3
3	Endocrine Dysfunction		0	1	2	3
4	Chronic Pain, Orthopedic Problems, Headaches		0	1	2	3
5	Depression		0	1	2	3
6	Anxiety		0	1	2	3
7	Anger		0	1	2	3
8	Hypervigilance		0	1	2	3
9	Posttraumatic Stress Disorder (PTSD)		0	1	2	3
10	Substance Abuse		0	1	2	3
11	Perceptual System Impairments (Hearing, Vision, Balance)		0	1	2	3
12	Cognitive Impairments (Concentration, Memory, Organization)		0	1	2	3
13	Marital and Family Concerns		0	1	2	3
14	Intimacy Concerns (Emotional, Sexual)		0	1	2	3
15	Military-Civilian Transition Difficulties		0	1	2	3
16	Toxic Exposure Illnesses and Cancers		0	1	2	3
17	Existential Concerns (Guilt, Loss, Grief, Moral Injury, Survivor's Guilt, Loss of Tribe)		0	1	2	3

Total sum score of all seventeen items: _____
Number of items scored above 2: _____

However, we must be wary of the PTSD disability trap. So far, half or more of all service members who ever served in Iraq or Afghanistan have been diagnosed and received lifetime PTSD disability cash payments from the VA. Yet, the best epidemiological evidence suggests the prevalence rate of PTSD in those who served in a war zone is only about 8 percent. In addition, most veterans who deployed were not combatants. This raises questions about how the PTSD diagnosis is being used by the large bureaucratic systems that care for service members and veterans.[3]

And here's one more thing about the VA system: despite the five billion dollars they spend every year on mental healthcare, they cannot or will not show any system-level administrative data on the effectiveness of their PTSD treatment programs. I've long been curious about this. I and other health advocates have asked but never received an answer. A common phrase I hear often from SOF veterans is that the VA's mantra is "medicate and isolate," suggesting that VA care is primarily about keeping veterans quiet rather than actually treating them.

What I consider to be the PTSD disability trap is the powerful systematic encouragement to become and remain a psychiatric invalid. For those who have experienced this pressure, I can only say the following: *Don't do that. Don't let that become your identity.* Remember that, with the right form of behavioral therapy, PTSD is a treatable condition. Consider as well the possibility that the diagnosis may even be inaccurate. For example, most operators don't have much of the fear reactivity required for the diagnosis.

---

3   See *Wounding Warriors: How Bad Policy is Making Veterans Sicker and Poorer* by Daniel Gade and Daniel Huang (Ballast Books, 2021)

"The VA System is a disability game, a total trap and life suck. A fool's errand."

—**Prime Hall**, former U.S. Marine Raider

Healthcare Needs That Are Unique, Not "Special"

Over the past decade I've often heard the argument—typically from neurologists, psychiatrists, psychologists, and military officers—that we must *not* develop treatment programs or services tailored specifically to the SOF community. The arguments invariably invoke the concept of "social justice" (i.e., we must have equal treatment for all) or a belief that PTSD is the primary problem and can be treated the same way it is among conventional soldiers and veterans. Often there is an unspoken undercurrent of judgment that the SOF community is seeking entitlement.

I counter with this: Yes, everyone who served in the military deserves to and absolutely should receive the effective care their injuries and impairments require. However, modern medical perspectives and care models for PTSD and traumatic brain injury (TBI) offered to operators by the Defense Health Agency (DHA) and the VA address only some of the parts, rarely the whole. SOF healthcare needs demand a comprehensive and multidisciplinary approach, delivered with a high level of awareness to SOF culture.

The "Establishment" Arguments
Against Operator Syndrome

There are powerful voices within mainstream medicine and among VA policy wonks that are circling their wagons to resist the framework of Operator Syndrome. I've heard this from a variety of sources, including those inside the VA, the DOD,

SOCOM, organized medicine, mental health professional associations, and several large veterans foundations. Some things are said openly, some are not.[4] Common arguments against Operator Syndrome—and my rejoinders—are as follows:

- "Operator Syndrome discriminates against those who were not in SOF; social justice requires treating all soldiers and veterans equally." My response: unique injuries require unique treatments.
- "It will stigmatize operators and harm recruitment and retention." My response: The specter of brain and orthopedic injuries does not appear to limit the number of athletes competing for roster spots on professional sports teams. Virtually every operator I've ever met has made it emphatically clear that even knowing what he knows now, he would still volunteer to do it all over again if he could.
- "It is not a 'real' diagnosis anyway." My response: that's correct—it is a whole systems framework to guide research, performance optimization, and treatment approaches for the unique injuries and impairments incurred by SOF.
- "It will require us to develop new programs and services." My response: Yes, it will. But that is no excuse to avoid providing quality medical care. Suck it up, because it's the right thing to do, and it supports our armed forces and national security.

---

4   In December 2022, I was permanently banned from LinkedIn for "misinformation" and "violation of community standards." Exactly why is unclear. In October and November, I had been blocked and scolded for posting links to published empirical medical studies documenting problems with the COVID mask mandates and vaccine. Then, in December, I reposted a message about resurgent Taliban atrocities under sharia law against women in Afghanistan. I was banned a few hours after that post.

Sadly, in medicine today, differences of opinion are often not settled with data, logic, and critical analyses. Too often, political ideologies in medicine not only trump empiricism, but actively censor it.

The VA and DOD are responsible for virtually all of the healthcare for veterans and service members. They hold the keys to a massive empire of medical treatments, facilities, pharmaceutical contracts, and specialized personnel. Moreover, these two federal departments represent powerful vested interests that hold a virtual monopoly on medical research pertaining to veterans and service members. Not only do they control what medical research may be conducted within their systems, but they also control almost all of the available research *funding*.

Although any medical scientist can apply for research grant funding from the National Institute of Health, this is not true with VA. Only VA employees are eligible to apply for VA research grants. You have to be in the club in order to play! The result of this is that VA medical researchers have *no competition* from scientists outside the system. This insularity leads to groupthink and a herd mentality. What's more, almost all medical research on veterans is conducted by a unionized workforce who must follow the political priorities of the VA's entrenched federal bureaucracy.

How could meaningful innovation not be stifled?

The PTSD "industry"—which includes Big Pharma and the VA's psychologists, social workers, and psychiatrists—is a behemoth. The Operator Syndrome framework runs counter to much of its accepted wisdom and standard practices. Powerful vested interests do not want to see the primacy of psychiatric treatments or branded psychotherapies downgraded. Small research empires would be disrupted. Career reputations would be threatened. Hospitals and clinics would need to retool. As a matter of fact, the current dominance of the entire mental health field would be diminished in favor of other medical disciplines.

All of this demonstrates how hard it is to find thoughtful, specialized healthcare services that meet the needs of the SOF community. As one active-duty SOF soldier told me recently: "*Nobody's coming for us.*" Many in the SOF community are aggressively exploring and adopting a wide range of nongovernmental solutions to their difficulties rather than waiting on and relying on the VA system.

Modern Healthcare: Fragmentation, Systems, and Insurance

Part of the problem that operators face—indeed, that we all face—is our current fragmented and highly specialized approach to medicine and healthcare. Rarely do specialists talk to one another, leading to broken communication when multiple health conditions are involved.

To meet the specific needs of the SOF community, a uniquely tailored, comprehensive, programmatic approach is almost certainly best. Intensive, multidisciplinary outpatient programs of two to eight weeks are likely the most effective format for providing this integrated care. Evaluation and treatment should address each of the conditions. The multidisciplinary team of medical and behavioral clinicians should routinely include neurologists, endocrinologists, sleep medicine specialists, physiatrists, psychiatrists, psychologists, orthopedists, gastroenterologists, physical therapists, pain medicine specialists, nutritionists, speech pathologists, vestibular medicine experts, internists, and other rehabilitation specialists.

The DOD has TBI-focused programs, known as the National Intrepid Center of Excellence (NICoE) and the Intrepid Spirit Centers, that provide comprehensive assessment for active-duty military personnel. However, these typically have long national waiting lists, are not specifically tailored to the unique needs of the SOF community, and are not available to retired military personnel. There are a small number of comparable programs on the civilian and veteran side, but they also have long waiting lists. Furthermore, while individual health insurance may cover some of the individual treatments needed, none that I know of currently cover the cost of uniquely tailored, comprehensive, multidisciplinary treatment programs for operators after they leave service.

Implications for First Responders and Other High-Risk Professions

The whole systems approach applied to military special operators may also be applicable to other high-risk professions, such as first responders. For example, in the course of their work, career firefighters face frequent sleep dysregulation or deprivation, personal danger, the deaths of comrades and civilians, and a high risk of traumatic brain injuries. Toxic environments from chemical, industrial, and residential fires can include smoke, benzene, toluene, carbon monoxide, natural gas, carbon dioxide, oxygen-deficient atmospheres, and potentially even the materials of the protective equipment worn. Obviously, all of this can cause profound and cumulative damage to the brain and every other bodily system. In fact, I and several colleagues recently proposed another whole systems framework for "Firefighter Syndrome."[5]

---

5   Christopher Frueh, et al, "'Firefighter Syndrome': A Proposed Whole Systems Framework," CRACKYL Magazine, August 2023.

Implications for Performance Optimization

While Operator Syndrome is a framework for understanding the downstream effects of a career in military special operations, it can also be used to structure efforts to mitigate these injuries during the active phase of a military career in order to maintain better health and sustain high performance. The need for this is intuitively obvious, if you think about it. I often coach or mentor active-duty operators in their twenties and thirties. We focus on maximizing approaches to diet, sleep, and recovery practices. I provide guidance on proactive medical testing (e.g., evaluation of hormone levels) and strategies to maintain and improve health across a wide range of domains. We engage strategies to maintain and improve marriages, parenting, and a performance mindset. Sometimes we address post-service career and life plans. In this way, the concepts and information contained in the book will have practical value for every stage of an operator's life, from initial selection to retirement or discharge, in midlife and beyond.

"Special Operators are expected to perform optimally while deployed in the most austere environments with the bare minimum when it comes to health and wellness resources. We spend more time and attention maintaining our equipment than we ever do maintaining ourselves. Our healthcare needs to match our level of performance and consider the environments we operate in. Conventional medicine is not meeting the standard."

—**Geoff Dardia**, functional medicine certified health coach, U.S. Army Special Forces Master Sergeant, founder of the SOF Health Initiative Program

Limitations of Medical Science

I acknowledge there are many scientific limitations to the information presented herein. Our medical paper about Operator Syndrome is a simple description of what I and many others have observed in our applied experiences with the SOF community. It was not a prospectively designed epidemiological or longitudinal research study. We have major scientific limitations in the form of knowledge gaps on how to fully understand the phenomena we term Operator Syndrome, including causative mechanisms. Moreover, we also know relatively little about how best to evaluate and treat TBI and many of the other associated specific conditions. With a primary focus on "mental health" in the current healthcare system, it seems unlikely that research enterprises are asking the right questions or looking in the right places.

Although we are faced with these limitations, uncertainty is no reason not to take action. Please consider this book to be my best, good-faith effort to provide education and practical guidance—based on what we now know—for operators and their spouses to more effectively care for themselves and their families. I also hope those who are not within the SOF community will learn something and perhaps even join efforts to help that community.

How to Use This Book

This is not an academic book. I did not write it for people with advanced healthcare degrees. For the most part, I have not footnoted or cited scientific references. My intention is for this book to provide a practical understanding of the Operator Syndrome framework and guidance on how operators and their spouses can pursue healing, recovery, and performance optimization.

Throughout the book, I have incorporated quotes from operators, spouses, and medical providers and scientists. Most of these quotes are personal statements provided by people I know—and, of course, are used with their permission. Some are quotes from the public statements or writings of others.

Now that you have completed reading Part One, you should have an understanding of the complex injuries, symptoms, and impairments that operators commonly experience.

Part Two is a series of short chapters that provide descriptions of and information on each of the conditions within the framework. These chapters conclude with concrete action steps that operators can take to review risk history, evaluate current status, reflect on lifestyle, and consider whether professional treatment is needed.

Part Three offers the good news: *Operator Syndrome conditions are highly treatable.* This section provides guidance, information, and strategies regarding medical treatments and lifestyle modifications that will help. *Make no mistake—there is every reason for hope*! (For quick reference, check the "Example Treatment Plan" at the end of Chapter 20.)

We have powerful therapies that can turn a life around and restore health, functioning, relationships, and quality of life. Of course, there is a place for traditional mental healthcare (including therapy, psychiatric medications). But there are also many other treatments not widely available or even commonly known about—including by experienced medical providers.

I believe that bilateral stellate ganglion block (SGB) treatment, ketamine infusion therapy, transcranial magnetic stimulation, and various psychedelic plant medicines all have the power to provide long-lasting relief from depression, PTSD, anxiety, anger, and insomnia. Each also probably improves cognitive functioning, relationships, and perspective on life itself.

We know SGB is very effective for treating some types of headaches as well as neck and shoulder pain. Ketamine and SGB used *in combination* may have synergistic effects, amplifying benefits.

Hyperbaric oxygen therapy, speech therapy, vestibular therapy, testosterone treatments, continuous positive airway pressure (CPAP) machines, peptide therapy, exome treatment, and stem cell therapy have all been game changers for many operators.

Many of us even believe (although with little research yet) that some of these treatments, especially in combination, may initiate neural plasticity—the growth of new neurons and dendrites, as well as the strengthening and development of pathways and connections in the brain. In other words, they may directly treat TBI at the most basic neuronal level. The overarching message of Part Three is this: physiological injuries can heal.

One last thing: This book can be read straight through like any other book, or you may turn directly to the chapter or sections of most interest to you. Most of the chapters will read as self-contained, short topical essays. From this point forward, unless otherwise indicated, my writing is addressed directly to operators.

Further Recommended Readings
* *A Message to Garcia* by Elbert Hubbard (1899)
* *The Warrior Elite: The Forging of SEAL Class 228* by Dick Couch (Crown, 2003)

- *Relentless Strike: The Secret History of Joint Special Operations Command* by Sean Naylor (St. Martin's Griffin, 2016)
- *All Secure: A Special Operations Soldier's Fight to Survive on the Battlefield and the Homefront* by Tom Satterly and Steve Jackson (Center Street, 2019)

PART TWO

THE CONDITIONS

CHAPTER 2

TRAUMATIC BRAIN INJURY

"'Operator Syndrome,' especially blast TBI (bTBI) and PTSD, are destroying the lives of special operators at an alarming rate."
—**Colonel Warren Stewart** and **Lieutenant Colonel Kevin M. Trujillo** in *Modern Warfare Destroys Brains: Creating Awareness and Educating the Force on the Effects of Blast Traumatic Brain Injury*

"I would have rather lost a limb than have to go to my third brain clinic. At least I would be able to see what exactly was wrong with me."
—**Daniel Luna**, EdD, U.S. Navy SEAL (Ret.)

"A career spent enduring concussive explosive blast wave after concussive explosive blast wave finally caught up with me. I started to suffer the many symptoms of what we now know were multiple minor traumatic brain injuries. Minor only in the sense that they didn't put me in a field hospital or emergency room like a gunshot wound, missing limb, or eye would have. I went through the extreme contrast of living a life of purpose as an elite performer in situations of life and death to having my life turned into so much

of a living nightmare that the only beneficial future I could imagine for my family was a future in which I ceased to exist. All this without a scratch on my body."

—**Andrew Marr**, MBA, U.S. Army Sergeant First Class (Ret.), 1ˢᵗ Special Forces Group, cofounder of Warrior Angels Foundation, board member and vice president of the Special Operations Association of America, author of *Tales from the Blast Factory: A Brain Injured Special Forces Green Beret's Journey Back from the Brink*

"For my entire time in the SEAL teams I was told that TBI and high-stress environments are bad for my health; however, no one explained what my body was going through—or suggested solutions. When I read 'Operator Syndrome' I was skeptical. It was only when I started to look at my life, my lab values, and my mental health that it all started to make sense. I had heavy bouts of depression and anxiety. My energy was lower than it ever had been. I didn't know what was wrong or who to turn to. All I was ever told was that I have PTSD and take these meds. There had to be a better way."

—**Joey Fio**, former U.S. Navy SEAL, senior director of health at the SEAL Future Foundation

"TBI isn't solely associated with combat. In fact, many service members I work with experienced the bulk of their brain injuries during training or as a result of toxic exposures. For these individuals the accumulation of repetitive injuries, few of which are given the conditions they need to heal, is like a slow boil with symptoms emerging and progressing over time. This makes it extremely difficult for service members and their teammates or families to know what is going on and why, let alone what to do about it."

—**Kate Pate**, neurophysiology PhD

"Upon exiting the military my husband had over forty document-ed concussive events during his twenty years of service. The path to healing and restoration was littered with confusion because of the myriad of issues that had accumulated during his career—and in large part had been ignored due to the incredibly high op-tempo that was required of Special Operators in the wake of 9/11."

—**Andrea Gallagher**, U.S. Navy SEAL spouse, president of the Pipe Hitter Foundation, founded with Eddie Gallagher

Traumatic brain injury—or TBI, for short—is one of the root causes of Operator Syndrome. Our brain is the primary organ of our nervous system, and along with the spinal cord, it makes up our entire central nervous system. Our brain organizes, processes, and directs the activities and processes of our body. This includes receiving, managing, and interpreting the information it receives from our sensory organs, like eyes and ears. It also includes using this information to direct messages that are sent to every other part of our body. This most precious part of us is carefully positioned within our skull, floating in cerebral spinal fluid (CSF) because it is fragile.

Our brain consists of the cerebrum, the brain stem, and the cerebellum, each containing a variety of areas and structures that have highly specialized functions. For example, if you damage the hippocampus, you might lose your memory; damage the amygdala, you might lose all fear; damage the paraventricular hypothalamus, you might eat yourself to death—literally eat to the point of bursting.

Brain injury, in other words, is no joke. TBI effects are usually general, spread around the brain, rather than highly specific to one small area. People with brain damage are likely to experience headaches, mood swings, personality changes, and cognitive impairments, especially with regard to memory, attention, and learning. They are also one and a half times more likely to misuse alcohol; two times more likely to be in fair or poor health; two and a half times more likely to be unhappy; and three times more likely to be disabled.

Our brain is delicate, and there are many ways to injure it, but for operators, brain damage comes in two primary forms.

Impact forces may occur, like being punched in the head or falling and landing on your head. These types of blows can cause concussions, which are bad enough in and of themselves, but the damage is also cumulative over the course of a lifetime. Postmortem brain studies have shown that some people with a history of many concussions developed a buildup of tau proteins that signals the presence of what is known as chronic traumatic encephalopathy (CTE).

Blast waves cause an additional type of brain damage. An explosion sends out waves of blast overpressure that will literally shear through the human body, damaging delicate tissues in the eyes, ears, lungs, and brains of everyone within the radius. Like impact forces, this type of damage is also cumulative. In 2016, a team of pathologists at Walter Reed National Military Medical Center conducted postmortem brain studies of a group of people who had had extensive blast wave exposure and showed substantial cognitive deficits before they died. These scientists found a pattern of scar tissue in the brain known as interface astroglial scarring.

There are also many other ways to injure the brain that don't involve concussions or blast waves, including heavy metal and other toxic exposures, night work and chronic sleep dysregulation, and substance abuse.

Combatants with traumatic brain injuries are likely to experience headaches, mood swings, personality changes, and cognitive impairments, especially in memory, attention, and learning. We also believe TBI is at least partially, if not primarily, responsible for hormonal imbalances, sleep apnea, insomnia, vestibular problems, depression, anger, and PTSD.

To put it another way: **TBI plays a major causal role in most aspects of Operator Syndrome**.

TBI, whether by impact force or blast wave overpressure, represents a massive invisible wound to the brain. Unfortunately, at this point in time, our scientific understanding of TBI is quite poor. We are in early days and still have so much to learn.

For one, we do not even know how to clinically diagnosis TBI or assess the damage. Brain neuroimaging like fMRI or PET scans is pretty nifty, but it rarely provides much usable clinical or diagnostic information. Neuropsychological performance testing—tests of attention, memory, IQ—can provide good information about functional deficits or impairments, such as to memory and concentration. Right now, however, only postmortem examination can really tell us about the damage inside the brain, and obviously, by then, it's too late to do anything about it. We also do not really know how to treat TBI. There is no magical pill or surgical procedure that will quickly and reliably repair your brain.

And yet, there are many things that can potentially help your brain heal and recover. These include formal medical treatments, such as hyperbaric oxygen therapy, hormone treatments, vestibular therapy, and speech pathology. In addition, you can possibly find help from stellate ganglion block therapy, ketamine therapy, other psychedelic compounds, transcranial magnetic stimulation, and psychotherapy. (These treatments will be reviewed in Part Three of this book.)

There are also many things you can do without medical care that can help your brain recover. Let's call the following lifestyle modifications or good health habits:

- Get lots of quality sleep and rest.
- Minimize use of alcohol, tobacco, and drugs.
- Eat a healthy diet with lots of protein, fruits, and vegetables.
- Consider dietary supplements of omega-3 and B vitamins.
- Get moderate and regular exercise.
- Engage socially with your family and friends.

An injured brain may not heal all the way or heal quickly, but natural recovery over time can really be quite significant. Unfortunately, because active operators are not typically afforded the opportunity for rest and recovery that is needed, natural recovery times are often interrupted.

———————

It is not really possible to provide you with a quick and simple questionnaire that will help measure the severity of your brain injuries or second- and third-order effects. You can, however, at least partially quantify the damages you may have sustained over the course of your life and career.

Most neurologists and other physicians diagnose TBI based on the discrete number of head injuries accumulated over the course of a lifetime and the extent of loss-of-consciousness

(LOC) events. However, this standard approach essentially struggles to minutely quantify blast wave exposures—including the small exposures that occur every time you pull a trigger—and all those so-called "minor" bumps to the noggin that occur regularly in training and on deployments.

Look at it this way: If you ever took a breacher course, trained as a sniper, or fired handheld rockets, then you have almost certainly injured your brain. You can be sure that jumping out of airplanes, combat diving, rappelling from helicopters, and hand-to-hand combat have not helped either.

———

Some Things You Can Do Right Now

Review your risk history using the questions and directives in the following sections:

TBI Diagnoses

1. How many impact force concussions have you sustained in your lifetime?
2. Have you ever been diagnosed with TBI?
3. Have you ever been evaluated for TBI?

Impact Force Injuries

Think back over the course of your entire life, including your childhood and all athletic activities. Make a list of every significant head injury—received in fights, falls, sports, vehicular or other accidents—that you can remember. Ask yourself:

1. Did you lose consciousness?
2. Did you receive any form of medical care afterward?

3. Did you experience headaches, dizziness, nausea, or confusion after the injury? If so, for how long?

Blast Exposures

We know that blast wave exposures cause a potentially sheering force through the brain and body. These exposures accumulate over time, but they are impossible to truly quantify in retrospect. Think about how many times over the course of your life you pulled a trigger, fired a rocket, or were near an explosion of any sort. Try to estimate how much total blast wave exposure you have had in your life. Be sure to consider it in relation to other people who are not operators.

Alcohol and Drug Use

1. Have you ever lost consciousness from an alcohol binge or drug overdose? If so, how many times?
2. What percentage of the total days of your adult life have you used alcohol and/or recreational drugs?
3. How many times in your life have you "binged" or consumed more than five standard drinks of alcohol?

Other Potential Brain Injury Exposures

1. How many nights in your life have you worked through the evening, until past midnight?
2. Have you ever lost consciousness from being "choked out"? If so, how many times?
3. How many parachute jumps have you made? How many hard landings?
4. How much combat diving experience have you had?
5. How much of the following have you had?

__heavy metal exposures __burn pits

__very loud noises __other toxic exposures

__night or late-shift work __riding small craft boats on rough waters

__rappelling from a helicopter __rucking with weight

Evaluate your current status. There are numerous neurobehavioral markers of TBI. Most of these can be more typically associated with health concerns not related to TBI, but the more of these that you have, the greater the likelihood that you may have TBI. Are you experiencing any of the following difficulties or impairments?

__frequent headaches __fatigue

__poor concentration __depression

__slow thinking __anxiety/PTSD

__poor memory __nausea or vomiting

__disorganization __light sensitivity

__indecisiveness __sound sensitivity

__unsteady balance __hearing loss

__blurry or double vision __tinnitus

__impaired hand-eye coordination __reduced finger dexterity

__tingling or numbness in your hands, feet, shoulders

Reflect on your lifestyle. Lifestyle modifications and habits can go a long way toward improving your brain health. Quality sleep (see Chapter 3), a healthy diet, moderate exercise, and an anti-inflammatory lifestyle (see Chapter 22) are all highly beneficial for your brain. It is also important to identify and reconsider any current activities that may cause further damage to your brain.

Consider whether you need professional treatment. Have you ever been formally evaluated for TBI? If not, you probably should seek out such an evaluation.

Final Thoughts on TBI

Remember, these are injuries. You are not "broken." You were injured in the course of your military service. Now it is time to give your brain a chance to heal and recover.

Further Recommended Readings

- *Tales From the Blast Factory: A Brain Injured Special Forces Green Beret's Journey Back from the Brink* by Adam Marr and Andrew Marr (Morgan James Publishing, 2018)
- *Modern Warfare Destroys Brains: Creating Awareness and Educating the Force on the Effects of Blast Traumatic Brain Injury* by Colonel Warren Stewart and Lieutenant Colonel Kevin M. Trujillo (Belfer Center: Harvard Kennedy School, 2020)

CHAPTER 3

SLEEP DISTURBANCE AND SLEEP DISORDERS

"As I left the Navy with several sleep issues (insomnia, hyper-vigilance, obstructive sleep apnea), one of my friends committed suicide. Ryan Larkin was a Navy SEAL sniper and medic and would never reach the age of thirty. What I realized is that Ryan suffered serious sleep-related issues. He used sedatives like Ambien and alcohol to fall asleep and stimulants to wake up. This is something that many of us did and was very common in the SEAL teams. What I didn't know then was how this 'pseudo sleep' wasn't as restorative as we hoped and that we would pay the price later. Ryan was awake for five days before he hanged himself in his parents' basement."

—**Robert Sweetman**, former U.S. Navy SEAL

"Throughout my career in special operations and multiple government programs, I developed severe sleep issues in conjunction with substance abuse. I rarely remembered dreams, but I often woke upset, scared, and disoriented. This past year after I met my girlfriend, she would lovingly look at me in the morning and explain what she saw. Her words were 'babe you fight a real war every

single night.' I was unaware that I was physically and emotionally fighting all night long. She told me I would end up on the floor applying a rear naked choke to a pillow, talk, yell, and cry. I didn't remember any of it but could feel the emotional toll daily. Since receiving stellate ganglion block and ketamine therapy I now sleep calmly through the night and awake without the added scares of my nightly battles."

—**Kevin Reeves**, former U.S. Army Ranger and Sniper, Air Force Pararescueman (PJ), private defense contractor

"Sleep makes you a better person, so make sure you sleep. No matter what or how, sleep is our #1. Talk about this and experiment. Try HBOT (hyperbaric oxygen therapy), blackout curtains, sound machines, different mattresses, or maybe even sleep separately. Just find what works for you both."

—**Leslie Luna**, U.S. Navy veteran, SEAL spouse

After a career in the U.S. Army, much of it with a Tier One special operations unit, Jason L. left the service and settled down with his high school sweetheart and their children. The family returned to their hometown and bought their dream house, situated on twenty acres. He was ready to live the quiet country life of a family man.

Or so Jason thought. There was a problem: he was exhausted all the time and had no energy or motivation. His wife was growing frustrated.

"Tell me about your sleep," I asked.

"I can't sleep for shit."

"How long does it take to fall asleep?"

"About twenty minutes if I've been drinking. A couple hours sober."

"Once you fall asleep, do you wake up before morning?"

"I wake up thirty minutes to an hour after I fall asleep. I always do. It's automatic, like clockwork. Then I'm in and out of sleep all night long until about 4 a.m. Eventually I just get up because I know I won't go back to sleep again."

His sleep was heavily fragmented, which meant he was not getting much REM or slow-wave sleep. I asked, "How many hours of sleep, in total, would you estimate that you get?"

"Maybe three, four hours a night. Unless I have a bad dream."

"Tell me about that."

"Couple times a week. It's impossible to predict. Sometimes I go weeks without one. Then I might have them every night for three or four nights in a row. Almost never remember them, but I wake up in a state of panic. Heart racing, breathing heavily, in a cold sweat, pillow is soaked and sheets are tossed around. Like I was wrestling a beast."

"Can you go back to sleep after that?"

He shook his head slowly. "I get up, splash cold water on my face, change my T-shirt, check the house, drink some water. After that I'll sit on the couch and watch some stupid TV. If I'm lucky, I fall asleep there until my wife shakes me. And I'll tell you this, she doesn't like it. She doesn't understand why I don't stay in bed. It's kind of personal for her."

I'd heard this sleep description before. It was a common pattern among operators. "How do you typically feel when you get up in the morning?"

"Completely drained."

———

Let's talk about sleep.[6] The reason we must consider sleep is that it's one of the critical aspects of life and survival for virtually every species of animal, and it is especially important for the health of our brains. Most of the operators I've met over the years have great difficulty sleeping, and many of them also have obstructive sleep apnea.

———————

We do not fully know why we sleep or all the mechanisms involved in it, but we do know it is incredibly important to our well-being. For example, if we do not allow our bodies meaningful episodes of sleep on a daily basis, our health and functioning deteriorate quickly. We need good sleep to consolidate memories and learning, restore and rejuvenate, grow muscle and repair tissue, and synthesize and balance hormones. During slow-wave deep sleep, our brains are able to clear out waste products via a glymphatic system that is only activated during this time. Our brain is quite active while we sleep. There is almost as much neural activity during sleep as there is when we are awake.

During the night, our brain cycles through two major types of sleep: non-REM and REM. Non-REM sleep involves high-amplitude, low-frequency electroencephalogram (EEG) rhythms, whereas REM—rapid eye movement—sleep is characterized by low-amplitude, high-frequency EEG rhythms. There are four stages of non-REM sleep that occur before we reach REM sleep.

The first state in a sleep cycle is light sleep, known as non-REM, stage 1. This is followed by deeper sleep in the forms of

———————

6   Portions of this chapter were previously published in an article titled "Best Sleep Habits to Optimize Performance, Wellness, and Longevity" that appeared in *Men's Journal* Everyday Warrior series in 2022.

non-REM stages 2 to 4, and then by a dream state referred to as REM sleep. A full sleep cycle lasts about ninety minutes the first time through and is usually repeated several more times every night, but with increasingly shorter cycles. If we are deprived of REM sleep, we will later produce more of it when allowed the chance. This is known as "REM rebound."

Each cycle of sleep has distinct neurorestorative processes. This means it is important not only to get a sufficient quantity of sleep every day, but also to get the quality of sleep your brain and body require. We need sufficient REM and slow-wave sleep on a nightly basis.

We should also talk about circadian rhythms. Circadian rhythms occurring in an environment free of natural time cues (e.g., living in a dark cave) stabilize at a little over twenty-four hours. At any given moment our degree of alertness depends, in part, on where we are in our circadian rhythm. People fall somewhere on a continuum, with "morning people" being on one end of the continuum and "evening people" being on the other, but this changes as we age. Young people tend to be either "evening people" or without preference, while older people (e.g., over sixty-five) are more typically "morning people." There is reason to believe that nocturnal lighting, especially the "blue" lights of computer screens and smart phones, have a disruptive effect on our circadian rhythms.

We don't know everything about sleep, but we do know for certain that getting sufficient amounts of quality sleep on a regular basis is a pillar of human health, well-being, and functional performance in just about every activity you can imagine.

All living animals sleep, but there is a wide range of sleep needs across species, with humans somewhat in the middle of that range. For example, horses (2.9 hours per day) and cows (3.9 hours per day) need very little sleep compared to cats (14.5 hours per day) and bats (19.9 hours per day).

Most humans need seven to nine hours of sleep at night for optimal health and performance. The quality of sleep is also important. There are both psychological and physical consequences associated with chronic sleep deprivation. Negative psychological and cognitive consequences include irritability, cognitive impairment, memory loss, impaired moral judgment, impaired judgment regarding risk-taking, impulsivity, restlessness, distractibility, poor concentration, depression, and, in acute situations, even hallucinations and paranoia.

The role of sleep in physical and medical health is also incredibly powerful. Chronic sleep deprivation contributes to impaired immune functioning, increased risk of type 2 diabetes, increased risk of heart disease, obesity, impaired psychomotor skills, and body aches and pains.

All of this is to say that both quantity and quality of sleep are absolutely critical for good health and maximum performance. Operators face a number of unique problems stemming from their military experiences that put them at special risk for problems with sleep. These include TBI, chronic headaches and body pain, endocrine dysfunction, psychological issues (e.g., depression, post-traumatic stress, survival guilt), nightmares, being "on guard" or hypervigilant at night, disrupted sleep schedules, and alcohol abuse. The prevalence of sleep disturbance among operators is about 85 to 98 percent, making it one of the most common areas of dysfunction—and one of the most serious health problems they face.

Common Sleep Disorders

Four sleep disorders common to operators are insomnia, sleep apnea, periodic limb movement disorder, and bruxism.

Insomnia is difficulty falling asleep, staying asleep, and an overall inability to get sufficient sleep. It is not defined by any specific number of hours of sleep because sleep needs vary widely among people. People with insomnia report difficulties sleeping *and* feeling chronically exhausted during their waking hours. This condition is nearly universal among operators.

Sleep apnea is a disorder of disrupted breathing during sleep. It is characterized by heavy snoring, periods of breathing cessation, and gasping for air. It is also accompanied by disruption of the normal sleep cycle, including slow-wave and REM sleep. Obstructive sleep apnea is very common among operators, likely related to blast exposures and years of high operational tempos that lead to chronic stress and elevated stress hormones (e.g., cortisol). This disorder can only be diagnosed by a polysomnography, a "sleep study," which involves spending the night sleeping in a special clinic while constant measurements are taken of breathing, brain wave activity, cardiac functioning, eye and limb movements, and body temperature. Sleep apnea is a severe disorder that can result in or contribute to numerous health conditions, including potential for heart attacks. It is usually treated with a CPAP machine.

Periodic limb movement disorder is related to restless leg syndrome and involves frequent jerking or kicking movements of the legs during sleep. Symptoms during waking hours can include a difficult-to-describe sensation in the legs, along with an irresistible urge to stretch, flex, or move them in some way. There are low-dose medications that can help manage this condition.

Bruxism is teeth grinding or jaw clenching while asleep. It causes headaches, jaw pain, and eventually cracked teeth that will require root canal treatment or extraction. Typically, treatment for bruxism is wearing a mouth guard throughout the night.

———

"Sleep hygiene" is a term used to describe optimal habits before, during, and after bedtime to help improve sleep quantity and quality. This list of behaviors (a.k.a. "dos and don'ts") includes:

Sleep Schedule
- It's important to keep a regular and consistent sleep schedule. Going to bed at about the same time every night may be the single most important sleep habit to develop. Go to bed about the same time every night; get up about the same time every morning.
- Avoid going to bed late and sleeping in on weekends.
- Limit daytime napping.

Sleep Environment
- At night your bedroom should be a sanctuary, set up in the following ways:
    - Very dark (though leave the shades cracked so some natural light is allowed to come in the morning)
    - Very quiet
    - Very cool (sixty-eight degrees is ideal for sleeping, as long as there are blankets on the bed)
- Be sure you have a comfortable mattress, bedding, and pillows.

- Do not run the television at night, and it is best to not even keep one in your bedroom.
- Do not keep a visible clock near your bed.
- Do not leave your phone within reach of your bed and do not leave its ringer on.

Other Habits

- Protect the time right before bed and develop a relaxing routine that includes the following:
  - Spend some quiet time with yourself immediately before going to bed. Listen to soothing music, meditate, pray, practice deep breathing, or read a calming book, though not in your bedroom.
  - Take hot showers or baths immediately before bed, which can change body temperature and prepare us for sleep.
  - For at least an hour or two before going to bed, do not do anything even slightly stressful or activating (i.e., do not pay bills, do not work, do not read emails, avoid conflict with your partner).
  - For at least an hour or two before going to bed, do not expose your eyes to light from a computer, tablet, or smart phone screen—the unique "blue" light these emit affects your eyes and brain in a way that impairs sleep. If you have to use these devices before bed, try using blue light glasses to counteract the effect.
- Use your bed for sleeping and sex only.
- Do not read or watch television in bed.
- If, after going to bed, you are awake for longer than twenty minutes or so, get up and do something relaxing

in another part of the house. When you begin to feel sleepy again, go back to bed. This strategy will help train you to sleep better in your bed.

- Do not watch a clock—in fact, as suggested above, do not even keep a visible clock in your bedroom.

- Consider using a sleep sound machine at night. Many people find that some type of constant, gentle noise in their sleep environment helps to block out other external sounds and lull them to sleep. Sleep sound machines typically provide a range of options, including "white noise," "rain," "babbling brook," "waves," "thunderstorm," and many others. According to a large survey conducted by Consumer Reports several years ago, sound machines were found to be one of the most effective strategies for promoting quality sleep. This can also help manage ringing in your ears (i.e., tinnitus).

Exercise

- Exercise regularly, preferably in the morning—but generally not after 2 p.m.
- Maintain a combination of regular aerobic and strength training for maximizing health and sleep.

Diet and Substances

- Do not use alcohol to help you sleep. Alcohol may seem to relax you, but it greatly interferes with the quality of sleep by impairing your brain's ability to go through the sleep cycles, leading to incidents of middle-of-the-night awakening, reduced REM sleep, and fragmented sleep overall.

- Avoid caffeine after midday. Late caffeine consumption impairs sleep for most people because it has a long half-life and stays in your system for up to twelve hours or more.
- Avoid nicotine products, if possible; they contribute to fragmented sleep.
- Avoid large meals close to bedtime.
- Eliminate or at least limit your consumption of soda, especially after midday.
- Eat a healthy diet.
  - Eliminate most sugar and processed foods from your daily diet.
  - Supplement your diet with fish oil (1,200 milligrams per day), magnesium (150 to 450 milligrams per day), and vitamin D3 (1,000 milligrams per day).

———

Sleep medications and supplements are widely used for insomnia, but most have significant side effects and limitations and should be generally used for only short periods of time. Many of these medications are addictive, cause balance problems, and can leave you groggy or cognitively impaired the next day. They can also interact dangerously with alcohol use. (Be sure to discuss use of supplements or medicine with a medical care provider.)

Supplements

Melatonin is a naturally occurring hormone produced by the pineal gland that helps to regulate sleep and wakefulness. It is involved in the entrainment (i.e., synchronization) of the circadian rhythms. As an over-the-counter supplement (in doses of three to ten milligrams), it can be useful for helping you fall asleep and also reducing the effects of jet lag when taken about an hour or two before bedtime. It appears to be safe for both short- and long-term usage, with few side effects. Some users note that it heightens the intensity of their dreams.

Magnesium is an important nutrient too often lacking in our diets. Many people find that taking magnesium (250 to 450 milligrams per day) two hours before going to bed helps them sleep better. There are also numerous proprietary products—typically blends of herbal extracts and vitamins—that may help. However, be aware that most of these products have not been rigorously studied.

Over-the-Counter Medications

Diphenhydramine (a.k.a. Benadryl) and doxylamine succinate (a.k.a. Unisom SleepTabs) are antihistamines commonly used to treat allergies, and they often have side effects of drowsiness that make them widely used for insomnia. In the 1980s and '90s, before hypnotic medications in current usage were developed and approved, diphenhydramine was frequently prescribed by physicians to treat insomnia. When used on a short-term basis, it appears to be effective for about two thirds of the population. However, *diphenhydramine is usually not recommended for people with TBI, because it may cause disturbances in memory and new learning.*

Prescription Medications

A variety of prescription medications are known to help with sleep, though most of these should not be taken every night for prolonged periods of time. Thus, caution is urged when considering use of any prescription medication. Perhaps the most commonly used medications that help people sleep are antidepressants, which do not cause dependence. The category of antidepressants used most often are SSRIs (selective serotonin reuptake inhibitors), which include Prozac, Paxil, Celexa, Lexapro, Zoloft, and Luvox. While these medications are general antidepressants, they often have a broad effect when used daily on improving sleep among people who are depressed or anxious. However, they do not work through causing drowsiness after being taken. Thus, even when taken in the morning, they can help improve nighttime sleep. Other antidepressants, such as trazodone and Elavil, do cause drowsiness and might be prescribed for sleep.

A category of antianxiety medications known as benzodiazepines, which include Valium, Xanax, Klonopin, and Ativan, also may be used to cause drowsiness and sleep, though for only shorter intervals due to their addictive properties (i.e., they cause dependence).

Finally, a category of medications known as "hypnotics" is approved specifically to treat insomnia. These include Ambien, Lunesta, and Sonata. These medications are effective for short-term use (two to six weeks) to help with sleep initiation, but are often not helpful in maintaining sleep through the night. Common side effects are headaches, next-morning grogginess (impaired cognitive and psychomotor functioning), and unusual sleep activities, including even sleep walking, sleep driving, and sleep eating! These medications are also associated with tolerance, dependence, and rebound insomnia after cessation of use.

Other Drugs

Although understudied and illegal in many states (and in the view of the federal government), there are anecdotal reports that marijuana (cannabis) helps people sleep and possibly manage chronic pain. Marijuana also has many other well-known, potentially adverse side effects and health consequences, and smoking anything is detrimental to pulmonary and cardiovascular health. CBD oil, a legal cannabis extract, provides no "high," but there is some limited evidence that it may help improve sleep, reduce anxiety, and reduce chronic pain.

Finally, there are many chemical compounds that may help induce sleep; however, virtually all of these will also affect the quality of your sleep, altering the way in which your brain naturally goes through the various sleep stages. Such disruptions to your sleep "architecture" may result in suboptimal amounts of restorative sleep (i.e., during slow-wave, REM stages).

———————

Some Things You Can Do Right Now

Consider your history of sleep while you were operating. Did you often work at night? Did you cross time zones frequently? How well did you sleep while you were operational? With regard to current sleep habits, ask yourself the following questions and discuss with your sleep partner, if you have one: How much sleep do you typically get at night? Do you often wake up throughout the night? Do you feel rested and refreshed in the morning? Has any sleep partner said that you snore heavily, stop breathing, or gasp for air while sleeping?

Evaluate your current status. Have you ever undergone a polysomnography (sleep study)? This is a medical procedure during which you spend the night in a sleep lab while a wide range of physiological processes are evaluated and monitored. These domains include breathing, pulse, blood oxygen, eye movements, limb movements, body temperature, and brain wave activity. If you have not had a sleep study before, or it has been more than five years, you should almost certainly request a referral for one. Primary care medical providers can order one for you. Additionally, it may help to wear a personal health tracker to learn more about your sleep and other associated patterns. The technology of modern trackers (e.g., Fitbit, Oura, Whoop, Suunto, Apple Watch, Garmin) and apps (e.g., Sleep Cycle) is pretty good these days. Not only can you learn how much total sleep you have gotten on any given night, including slow-wave and REM sleep, you can also usually see graphs detailing the night's sleep that show you when you were in the various stages of sleep or consciousness. This data can be very useful.

Reflect on your lifestyle. Consider what you can do to improve your "sleep hygiene"—and then do it. Use the bullet-pointed guides above to help.

Consider whether you need professional treatment. If you have not had a sleep study, you should ask for one—and then you should follow the treatment recommendations. A lot of guys complain about using a CPAP, and I get it: using a CPAP is a hassle, it can feel restrictive, and it may interfere with physical intimacy. But guess what? It may also offer profound benefits to the quality of your sleep, which in turn may lead to profound benefits to your brain, cognitive functioning, emotional states, and many other aspects of your overall health. For many operators it can be an incredible game changer.

Final Thoughts on Sleep

I strongly encourage you to prioritize your "Zs." It may be the most important thing you can do for your overall health, wellness, and functioning.

Further Recommended Readings

- *The Sleep Solution: Why Your Sleep Is Broken and How to Fix It* by W. Chris Winter, MD (Berkeley, 2017)
- *Why We Sleep: Unlocking the Power of Sleep and Dreams* by Matthew Walker, PhD (Scribner, 2017)

CHAPTER 4

HORMONAL DYSFUNCTION

"I have the testosterone of an eighty-year-old man."
> —**Anonymous** (age forty-two), private defense
> contractor and former U.S. Marine Corps Scout
> Sniper (serving twenty-one years combined)

"Throughout the military, and specifically the SEAL Teams and other Special Operations units, undiagnosed endocrine disorders, including low testosterone, are more and more common. Whether it be the chemicals that we are exposed to throughout our careers, daily life, or the obvious chronic stressors associated with the job itself, an all-out assault has been waged on our endocrine system. Through different lines of effort by academia and the hobbyist alike, special operators are able to protect and rebuild one of their most precious resources: their testosterone. This precious molecule will inevitably aid in the protection of the individual, and the nation that he or she swore to protect."
> —**Sean Teel**, U.S. Navy SEAL

"In my clinical experience, the primary symptoms that lead to operators seeking help are symptoms associated with endocrine dysfunction. Testosterone, growth hormone, thyroid, cortisol, epinephrine, and norepinephrine have strong associations with one's ability to sleep, focus, control emotions, communicate effectively, maintain muscle mass, burn fat as a fuel source, exercise intensely, and recover from exercise, among others."

—**Kirk Parsley**, MD, former U.S. Navy SEAL, physician to the SEALs

Show me a military special operator with low testosterone and I'll show you a man who is tired, distractible, irritable, and depressed. He is not sleeping very well, cannot concentrate, has little motivation to work out or do much of anything, has low sex drive, and is experiencing changes to his muscle mass and body composition. He often experiences erectile dysfunction and is embarrassed about it. His bone density health may be at risk. He wonders what has happened to him and why he has changed so much—and in so many different ways—compared to when he first joined the military. If he has elevated estrogen, he may also develop gynecomastia (enlarged male breast tissue often derogatorily referred to as "man boobs").

I and many others have come to believe that low testosterone is an inevitable outcome for virtually every operator, if they serve long enough. Many operators are discovering hormonal abnormalities within a few years after completing selection and training.

But why? Unfortunately, no one knows precisely why. However, I think the following equation provides a very broad, imprecise explanation:

TBI + high op tempos with chronic stress + chronic sleep deprivation or dysregulation + heavy metal exposures = hormonal dysfunction

Of course, the conditions and symptoms above are part of the reality of being an operator—and as a consequence, so is hormonal dysregulation, for most.

In my conversations with operators, I usually ask a simple series of questions: "Have you ever had a blood test specifically to evaluate your hormonal functioning? If so, how recently? What did the test(s) show? Have you ever or are you now receiving endogenous testosterone or other medications to address hormonal dysregulation?"

Several years ago, the operators I spoke with did not have much awareness of their testosterone levels. Many were surprised to hear that it might be a problem for them, but now, many operators seem to know they should be tracking their testosterone.

Anecdotally, I estimate that about 80 percent of the operators I speak with either have medically diagnosed low testosterone or have testosterone that is low, but not quite low enough to result in a diagnosis. Of the other 20 percent, many have never been tested or have not been tested in the past five years.

It is important to remember that modern medicine does not compare an operator's testosterone to their own personal baseline (e.g., their testosterone level at age eighteen), but to that of other men from the "general population." Thus, it is possible that even when an operator is told his testosterone is "normal" or "okay," it may be dramatically lower than it previously had been.

Low testosterone is a very common and significant problem for operators. Unfortunately, it is rarely evaluated or treated by most mental health clinicians, and many physicians in both the VA and DOD are reluctant to treat it.

————————

Our endocrine system is a complex messenger system within our body that includes all of our glands and hormones. Glands release hormones into the bloodstream; hormones are chemicals that influence and direct our moods, cognitive functioning, behaviors, and even our anatomy. The endocrine system starts in the brain with the hypothalamus, a structure which controls the pituitary gland and connects the endocrine system to the nervous system. The pituitary is the "master gland" of the endocrine system. It regulates the thyroid, parathyroids, pineal body, thymus, adrenal gland, pancreas, and sex organs (ovaries for females; testes for males).

Endocrine hormones include adrenaline (or epinephrine), testosterone, estrogen, progesterone, insulin, glucagon, growth hormone, melatonin, oxytocin, vasopressin, prolactin, thyroid-stimulating hormone, calcitonin, corticosteroids, erythropoietin, and many others. Some hormones are also neurotransmitters. For example, epinephrine and adrenaline are the same chemical compound. We call it epinephrine when it functions as a neurotransmitter (i.e., sending messages in the nervous system) and adrenaline when it is released into the bloodstream.

These glands and hormones work closely with our nervous system, circulatory system, digestive system, and every other system in our body to help regulate and manage many of the biological processes in our bodies throughout our lifespan. They operate on a circadian cycle and quality sleep is critical for them to function optimally.

So, what can a man do if he has low testosterone?

Lifestyle modifications can help restore depleted testosterone levels for many. This means lots of rest, sleep, and recovery (which are difficult, if not impossible, to obtain while an operator is on active status). Eating a quality diet is also critical. Focus on grass-fed, organic meats, eggs, and dairy. Eat lots of vegetables, fiber, and healthy fats. Be sure to get plenty of vitamins B and D, zinc, selenium, and magnesium. Drink your water; stay hydrated. Eliminate or reduce fast food, junk food, processed food, soda, and added sugar.

Simply put: your aim should be to live an anti-inflammatory lifestyle (for more on this, see Chapter 22).

In addition to the above, medical treatment may be necessary. This means that regular supplementation of exogenous testosterone (i.e., testosterone replacement therapy, or TRT) may be necessary for some operators. It is typically delivered via injections, pellets, patches, or gels. However, be aware that this form of treatment is not necessarily effective or appropriate for everyone and comes with potential risks, such as worsening sleep apnea, acne, rashes, reduced fertility, prostate cancer, overproduction of red blood cells and blood clots, and increased risk for heart attacks, strokes, or pulmonary embolisms. Generally, once TRT is started, it is a long-term, or even lifelong, treatment.

Some Things You Can Do Now

Review your risk history. If you ever trained or functioned as a military special operator, you are at a very high risk for low testosterone and other hormonal dysregulations.

Evaluate your current status. Answer the questions I mentioned earlier in this chapter: Have you ever had a blood test specifically to evaluate your hormonal functioning? If so, how recently? What did the test(s) show? Have you ever or are you now receiving endogenous testosterone or other medications to address hormonal dysregulation?

Decide if you need professional treatment. If you have not had your hormones tested within the past few years, you should ask a primary care provider to refer you for the necessary blood test.

Final Thoughts on Hormonal Dysfunction

Low testosterone and other hormonal dysregulations represent one of the signature injuries faced by operators. Low testosterone causes both suffering and functional impairments. Too often, it goes unrecognized, undiagnosed, and untreated. Do not let this happen to you. If you haven't already done so, ask a primary care provider to conduct the necessary blood tests.

CHAPTER 5

CHRONIC PAIN AND HEADACHES

"I live with constant chronic joint pain. No operator will come out of a career in special operations without having to manage through chronic, lifelong pain. While the journey is absolutely worth it, it is a part of the cost of this level of service."
—David Dezso, former U.S. Army Special Forces

"The day-to-day pain from multiple injuries, arthritis, and the inflammation hurt for many, many years while in the SEAL teams and long after as well. The pain that puts a hurting on me is my lower lumbar injury from wrecking my combat dune buggy, a.k.a. DPV, prior to invading Iraq in March of 2003. The worst pain was my TBI migraines from explosive breaches, shooting rockets, automatic weapons, etc. There are THOUSANDS of times that I wanted to slam a hatchet into my skull thinking it would give me some relief!"
—Johnny Sotello, former U.S. Navy SEAL

"As a retired Special Warfare Boat Operator (SWCC), I have had eleven joint surgeries, three fractured vertebrae, seven bulging discs—all discs are compressed—and many other orthopedic

injuries. I endured over one million high G-force wave pounding events on SWCC fast boats, causing hundreds of thousands of mT-BIs, leading to a nexus of post-concussion syndrome. I can account for twenty-five different symptoms of TBI. I have depression, anxiety, sleep apnea, insomnia, neurocognitive disorder and many other issues that can be found within the 'Operator Syndrome' umbrella. In my ongoing research over the last three years, every retired SWCC operator I have talked with has the majority of issues that I do."

—**Michael "Anthony" Smith**, U.S. Navy Special Warfare Combat Crewman (Ret.)

"Pain pills are only a temporary option and never to be looked at as a permanent solution. Alternate methods like CBD, plant medicines, stem cell, and eastern medicine practices are what I have seen that has worked the best for long-term pain management. Plants mixed with breath practice, water, and movement is the answer for a sustainable quality of life. Stem cell changed the game for me. I had stem cell IV in Mexico and my lower back has been strong since that procedure three years ago. I am a true believer in stem cell because before that, I tried everything the VA gave me, burned my nerves off around the L5 S1 disc, did meds for years, physical therapy for a decade…nothing worked until stem cell."

—**Prime Hall**, former U.S. Marine Raider

Military special operators put a lot of miles on their body. Running, rucking, rappelling, swimming, diving, and jumping—usually while carrying a hundred pounds or more—are an inherent aspect of the job, along with incurring numerous blast exposures and impact forces to the head.

This is obvious to anyone familiar with this specialized service. It is equally obvious that chronic orthopedic pain and headaches related to TBI must be common among operators—which they are.

When I ask an operator if they have any chronic pain, I very often receive the following answer: "*Every joint in my body.*" (Often this sentiment is expressed in more colorful ways.)

Virtually every operator I have spoken with acknowledges that he lives with chronic pain, and many have severe headaches. But this pain is often dismissed by the sufferers as something that runs in the "background" and can be ignored. "I've hurt worse" or "other guys hurt a lot worse than me" are common sentiments. Many guys accept this pain as something they simply have to live with. They may not tell their medical providers or even their partners about it.

During their military service, operators will often not admit it when they are injured. They may not ask for help. Assessment and treatment of injuries takes time away from training and may mean missing a deployment or operating under restrictions.

Like cats, operators hide their pain and push through it as though nothing is wrong. They cannot afford to be seen as "weak" or too impaired to function effectively.

Operators do not want to let their teammates down. They do not want to be taken out of the fight. They do not want their families to worry. Chronic, nagging injuries are accepted as part of what the job means, and consequently, they can never be an operator's reason to cease giving full effort. This becomes a cultural moral code that is deeply internalized.

Stoicism—as represented in writings of the ancients (e.g., Marcus Aurelius)—is a terrific philosophical approach to this world. But you can be stoic about pain and also seek ways to eliminate or manage it.

Modern medicine is not very good at pain management. Orthopedic surgeries can correct many functional injuries, eventually resulting in reduced pain, but too frequently some pain continues after surgery. Opiates can help manage pain in the short term, but they also carry vicious risks of side effects and addiction. Stay wary of long-term painkiller use. Physical therapy, massage, and chiropractic treatments can all help in lieu of opiates. Cognitive behavioral therapy for pain management is also a powerful approach. Stellate ganglion block therapy and specific medications or injections may help reduce or eliminate headaches, including migraines.

Medical treatment is unlikely to be a full solution for chronic pain. Lifestyle modifications and habits must be part of the solution. Toward this end, ask yourself the following questions: What is your current workout regimen? Are you training smartly? Are you training for the right mission? Remember, if you are no longer on active duty, you are now training for a very different mission, one aiming for good health, longevity, and mobility. Too many operators continue to work out with the same intensity as when they were young soldiers.

That is *no bueno*. I'm not a personal trainer, but here are my thoughts:

1. Strength training is critically important, but free weights and body-weight calisthenics are very hard on ligaments and tendons. Risk of significant injuries is high. My suggestion is to switch entirely to variable resistance bands. I suggest using the large, flat bands (like giant rubber bands) instead of the hollow

tubes with handles. If you combine these large bands with a shoulder-width Olympic bar and a plate (to thread the bands under), you can achieve an amazing strength-training workout. Variable resistance bands work with your natural strength curve, instead of against it as free- and body-weight exercises do. They are easiest in the unstretched position—when you are at your weakest point. As you push or pull through the range of motion, the bands stretch, and the resistance increases in proportion with your strength curve. You can also go to complete failure and then continue with partial reps. This is very gentle on your joints, and you may find that some of your joint pain disappears naturally over time.

2. Past a certain point in life, running is not your friend. It is hard on the knees, back, ankles, and other joints. Better to minimize or eliminate running altogether, replacing it with lower-impact forms of cardio—walking, swimming, ellipticals. You should probably also aim for a greatly reduced amount of cardio—about three hours a week total should be plenty for most guys. If you use a high-intensity interval training (HIIT) or Tabata approach, then you can spend much less time doing cardio.

3. Stretching, or a practice like yoga, can be an important addition to a healthy conditioning program.

4. There are other practices that may help with pain and headaches. Anything that reduces chronic systemic inflammation is likely to be beneficial: hot sauna bathing, meditation, an anti-inflammatory diet, quality sleep, etc. Float tank therapy, also known as sensory

deprivation, removes spinal compression for a period of time while you float in a pitch-dark, soundproof tank filled with a foot of salt water. This can induce a deep state of relaxation and may improve mood, cognition, and pain.

Some Things You Can Do Now

Review your risk history. What is the total "mileage" on your body compared to other men your age? How many orthopedic surgeries have you had? What types of rehabilitation therapies have you tried in the past?

Evaluate your current status. What hurts now? When does it hurt? How much does it hurt? How long does it hurt for? How do headaches and pain impair your ability to function or sleep? What would you like to do that you are unable to? What helps reduce or manage the pain?

Consider lifestyle factors. Be honest with yourself. Are there orthopedic surgeries you have put off? Is your current workout regimen compounding your injuries and pain? What lifestyle changes can you make that might help?

Decide if you need professional treatment. If you are living with chronic pain or headaches, seek solutions—medical care, lifestyle modifications, specific therapeutic practices, or some combination of all three.

Final Thoughts on Chronic Pain and Headaches

Operators incur enormous damage to their joints and heads over the course of their careers. This includes both acute and gradual injuries. Chronic pain and headaches are inevitable, but there are many potential solutions.

Further Recommended Readings

- *The Song of Our Scars: The Untold Story of Pain* by Haider Warraich (Basic Books, 2022)
- *The Way Out: A Revolutionary, Scientifically Proven Approach to Healing Chronic Pain* by Alan Gordon and Alon Ziv (Avery, 2022)

CHAPTER 6

DEPRESSION

"The cumulative effects of a severe TBI and many mild brain injuries made me struggle with basic tasks. I still performed well enough to be useable, but my performance was less than the average operator. The consequences of these injuries, as well as a lack of awareness, left all the weight of responsibility entirely on my perceived lack of capability, contributing to depression, anger, and substance abuse."

—**Chad White**, U.S. Army Sergeant First Class
(Ret.), 3rd Special Forces Group

"After my time in the teams, I found myself in a depressive state for the first time in my life. This despite being 'successful' with a great job, good education, and loving family. I now know I was suffering because I lost my team and purpose."

—**Jonathan D. Wilson**, former U.S. Navy
SEAL, cofounder and former CEO of the SEAL
Future Foundation, cofounder and CEO of INVI
Mindhealth

"By nature, SOF personnel are forced to build coping mechanisms to mute the extreme emotional highs and lows that come with the job. Being able to perform well in a high-stress or high-threat environment is mandatory, as is dealing with loss—from losing a teammate in combat to separation from family and home. The consequences of bottling these emotions over time can be severe and are something that many SOF combat veterans face for years beyond the action."

—**Ryan Land**, former U.S. Army Special Forces

"Not everyone that suffers symptoms of TBI/depression have problems with alcohol and/or drugs, though many do. I compensated for my undiagnosed symptoms of TBI/depression by overeating. Overeating is a terrible and vicious spiral. Exactly like alcohol and/or drugs, it makes the TBI/depression worse. The more depressed I got, the more I craved 'bad' food for 'comfort.' The more overweight I got, the more depressed I became. The more overweight, the worse my health was. It's vicious and unrelenting."

—**Darrell Utt**, U.S. Army Special Forces (Ret.)

Major depressive disorder is a relatively common psychiatric condition. It is also potentially a life-threatening illness, because it is one of the primary causes of suicide. The World Health Organization identifies clinical depression as a leading cause of disability worldwide and a major contributor to the overall burden of disease around the world. It harms the individual, their family, and all of society.

Symptoms of depression include the following:

- Sadness, hopelessness
- Anger and irritability
- Sleep disruption
- Anhedonia (loss of pleasure and enjoyment)
- Fatigue and low energy
- Emptiness, low motivation
- Appetite changes and weight gain or loss
- Social isolation
- Difficulty concentrating
- Physical symptoms (pain, headaches, gastrointestinal distress)
- Suicidality

Depression is sheer misery. It involves emotions (e.g., sadness), cognitions (e.g., pessimistic thoughts, hopelessness), behaviors (e.g., social withdrawal, reduced activity), and physical reactions (e.g., reduced immune functioning). It also leads to impairments in general functioning.

Other mood disorders can include persistent depressive disorder (also known as dysthymia), postpartum depression, and bipolar disorders I and II. These are serious conditions as well, but they are not as common as major depressive disorder.

Depression is a condition that affects people from all walks of life, and it can be caused by many things, although a primary risk factor is a family history of depression. If your parents, grandparents, or siblings have struggled with depression, you are more likely to as well. In other words, depression has a very strong genetic component to it.

Depression can also be caused by more immediate problems such as chronic stress, loss and grief, psychological trauma, and certain medical conditions. For example, men with low testosterone often appear to be severely depressed, but instead of Prozac or other antidepressants, they need testosterone supplementation in order to feel better. Medical illnesses such as heart disease or diabetes often contribute to depression.

Why are operators prone to depression? Part of the answer is that depression, anxiety, and PTSD typically go together—one great big bucket of psychological desolation. Other contributing factors to their depression may include chronic pain, sleep deprivation, social isolation, loss of purpose, TBI, marital discord, and grief—all common aspects of an operator's transition experience after military service.

Also, remember: alcohol is a "depressant." It might help you feel better for a few minutes or hours, and it might help you fall asleep, or pass out, but over time it depresses your nervous system and fragments your sleep, disrupting the various sleep phases and leaving you exhausted and wretched the next morning. Over time, heavy alcohol use can make depression worse.

There are differences in the manifestation of depression between the sexes. Women with depression are likely to experience overwhelming sadness and cry more. Men with depression are more likely to experience emptiness and anger. Women, encouraged by societal gender norms, are more likely than men to talk about their emotions and to seek treatment. Men are more likely to socially isolate, to abuse alcohol or drugs, and to attempt to distract themselves with work. Statistically, females are much more likely to attempt suicide, but males are much more likely to succeed in suicide attempts, primarily because they use more mechanically lethal means, such as firearms.

When we talk about depression, we also have to talk about suicide. People suffering from severe depression are at considerable risk of dying by suicide. As a result, depression is potentially a life-threatening illness, and a small but significant percentage of sufferers kill themselves. Recent losses, humiliations, or rejections can amplify this risk.

The good news is that we have many different forms of effective treatments for depression. Traditional treatment for depression has been psychotherapy and psychiatric medications, and the past decade has brought major advances in other lesser-known therapeutics.

Psychotherapy is a powerful intervention. There are different schools of thought regarding which modes of therapy work best, and many of these variations have been studied extensively. The good news is that talking therapies that focus on emotions, cognitions, or behaviors can all help alleviate symptoms and lead to remission, or even a long-standing cure.

Psychiatric medications are generally safe and nonaddictive, and most have minimal side effects for most people, even over many years of use. The largest category of antidepressant medications are SSRIs (selective serotonin reuptake inhibitors, a name that describes the neuronal mechanism of action). These include fluoxetine (Prozac), sertraline (Zoloft), citalopram (Celexa), escitalopram (Lexapro), and others. Keep in mind that you and your prescribing doctor will not immediately know which antidepressant medication will work best for you, meaning there will be a process of "trial and error" that can potentially take months.

Brain stimulation therapies are now shown to be effective for many people with depression, including an FDA-approved treatment called transcranial magnetic stimulation (TMS). It involves about thirty sessions (twenty to thirty minutes each, spread over six to ten weeks), during which magnetic fields target the brain with very low doses of energy. This is a safe and effective treatment—and it may also offer some relief from symptoms of TBI. Another form of brain stimulation used for depression is electroconvulsive treatment (ECT), which has been administered in the same way for over eighty years. ECT uses electric currents to induce brief seizures in patients, and it is considered to be a relatively safe and effective treatment specifically for people with severe, treatment-resistant depression (i.e., they have tried everything else in the psychiatric toolkit).

Ketamine is a synthesized hallucinogenic compound often used as a recreational drug, but it has also been widely prescribed in medicine for over fifty years as a dissociative anesthetic and painkiller. In addition, it is FDA-approved for treatment of depression. Ketamine can be delivered in a variety of ways, but intravenous infusion is recommended. Like TMS, this is a safe and effective treatment—and it may also offer benefits for symptoms of TBI. (And yes, ketamine is also used in veterinary medicine.)

Psychedelic compounds other than ketamine also show great promise for treating major depressive disorder and the symptoms that often go with it. In the U.S., a growing body of research supports the use of MDMA and psilocybin. Numerous randomized controlled trials (the "gold standard" of medicine's research methodology) have demonstrated significant efficacy for these two compounds, and both are nearing

FDA approval. Pioneering work conducted in Mexico and other countries outside the U.S. demonstrates perhaps even larger benefits from ayahuasca, ibogaine, and 5-MeO-DMT.

Lifestyle habits also make a big difference in preventing or reducing symptoms of depression. Regular, moderate **exercise** is one of the most powerful antidepressants known to man. Take a brisk walk, push or pull some weights or other resistance, and stretch. Many operators find that yoga, jiujitsu, or even salsa dancing are nice additions to their workouts. An **anti-inflammatory diet** is also very important, emphasizing vegetables, fruits, whole grains, lean meats, seafood, quality fats, beans, and seeds. Cook at home with whole foods, using the rainbow of fresh fruits and vegetables. Be sure to get plenty of protein. Avoid highly processed foods, including fast foods, junk foods, packaged baked goods, and added sugars. These are all inflammatory and consequently terrible for you! They can cause damage to your brain, mood, energy level, cognitive functioning, and joint health. (And yes, it should be apparent by now that I'm in the camp of those who believe sugar and processed foods are poison.)

Rest and recovery habits are imperative. Good sleep hygiene is a must. Additionally, engage in other soul-filling activities: meditation, prayer, church, social activities, cooking, intimacy, sex, hobbies, listening to or performing music, writing, or some daily pursuit of mission and purpose. Hop in a sauna. Research shows that taking a hot sauna bath three times a week is a powerful antidepressant!

Bottom line: If you are suffering from depression, please seek help, because this is a treatable condition—and treatment might just save your life. Most of the treatments for depression are also likely to provide relief from symptoms of anxiety, depression, anger, and insomnia. Keep in mind that there are many solutions out there. None of them work for everybody, so treatment and rehabilitation take time and a willingness to try different interventions.

Some Things You Can Do Now

Review your risk history. Do you have a family history of depression? Have you ever been diagnosed with or treated for depression? Are you prone to bad moods? Pessimistic thinking?

Evaluate your current status. Are you currently feeling depressed? How many of the symptoms above do you have, and how severe are they? Do people who know you well think you are depressed?

Consider lifestyle factors. Consider whether your lifestyle is anti-inflammatory. Do you exercise, eat, and sleep as you want to? Do you have regular social contact with people you care for and trust? Do you use drugs or alcohol to self-medicate?

Decide if you need professional treatment. If you have severe symptoms of depression or are feeling suicidal, you should probably seek treatment.

Final Thoughts on Depression

Depression is a disease of despair and a life-threatening illness, but it is treatable. If you are depressed, ask for, seek out, and find the therapeutics that will help you. They are out there.

CHAPTER 7

ANXIETY

"I was out of the military for about a year when I had my first anxiety attack, having no idea what was happening to me. I was in Target and took a turn down the lightbulb aisle. The intensity of the lights and flashing triggered a reaction that sent a wave of emotions across me. These emotions mimicked what I had felt overseas in combat. I reflect back on the countless deployments, the close calls, and that it was the light bulb aisle at Target that sent me down the path of my first anxiety attack."

—**Jonathan D. Wilson**, former U.S. Navy SEAL, cofounder and former CEO of the SEAL Future Foundation

"Understanding what produces anxiety in him still perplexes me at times. I've observed most people display anxiety during busy seasons of life or when overwhelmed. For him, stillness is an anxiety driver. Supporting him through new sources of stimulation has looked like everything from going for multiple midday walks to us becoming first-time boat owners."

—**Corrie Burton**, U.S. Army Special Forces fiancée

Everyone feels anxious from time to time. This is a normal part of the human experience. Anxiety is an adaptation, a survival strategy. It is our nervous system's way of helping our bodies respond instantaneously to environmental threats. It motivates us to act and, up to a certain point, helps enhance performance; however, beyond a certain point of severity, it impairs performance. (If you want to nerd out a little, look up the Yerkes-Dodson Law, which considers the empirical relationship between anxiety and performance.)

Anxiety is "turned on" by the autonomic nervous system, a division of the central nervous system. Your autonomic nervous system has three divisions—the sympathetic, parasympathetic, and enteric. These subdivisions work in harmony with each other. Most of the time our parasympathetic nervous system is quietly running, monitoring, and regulating the various systems and processes in our body. This includes breathing, digesting, pumping blood, and many other biological processes.

Once in a while we may become aware of a danger or a threat in our environment. When this happens, our sympathetic nervous system takes over. It kick-starts the release of adrenaline and cortisol, instantly raising our respiration and pulse rates, reallocating resources from our gut and the central parts of our bodies out to our extremities. This is often known as the "fight or flight" response.

As humans, we have a very sensitive and finely tuned nervous system on constant alert for threats. Although this system evolved to help us survive as a species, our technology has outpaced our biological evolution. Modern humans face far more choices and enormous complexities compared to our ancestors and the simple lives they lived. Sometimes our physiological responses are out of alignment with the nature and severity of potential threats.

There are a number of common anxiety-based psychiatric disorders. Phobias, social anxiety disorder, obsessive compulsive disorder, panic disorder, PTSD, and general anxiety disorder.

Many operators go through anxious periods during which they experience some of the symptoms of general anxiety.

Symptoms of general anxiety include:

- Anxiety, nervousness
- Uncontrollable worry
- Catastrophic thinking
- Constant muscle tension
- Inability to relax
- Dread that something terrible might happen
- Irritability
- Indecisiveness
- Difficulty concentrating
- Insomnia and fatigue
- Physical symptoms (pain, headaches, gastrointestinal distress)

A key point about anxiety: Humans are *all* more susceptible to anxiety when we are in pain, sleep-deprived, helpless, suffering effects of TBI, under chronic or acute stress, or going through major life transitions.

Think about a soldier getting out of military service, trying to establish a new career and family life. Now think about that soldier doing it with years of chronic stress, sleep deprivation, brain and orthopedic injuries, chronic pain and headaches, hormonal imbalances, sleep disorders, cognitive impairments, and medical conditions—all layered on top of the demands of civilian life.

Sound familiar? It is perfectly normal to be regularly anxious if you are an operator.

The good news is that anxiety is highly treatable, even more so than depression. Professional treatments such as cognitive behavioral therapies (CBT) are usually time-limited, accessible, and very effective. Exposure-based therapies that involve talking or journaling about stressful experiences or anxieties are usually the psychotherapy of choice for anxiety. Mindfulness approaches can help you live in the moment. (Antidepressant psychiatric medications may be prescribed and can help somewhat, but they are rarely a long-term effective solution for anxiety.)

We also know there are many lifestyle habits and therapeutics that can help reduce anxiety, including meditation, prayer, sleep hygiene, exercise, talking with friends, float tank therapy, relaxation exercises, yoga, stretching, walking in nature, and many other practices. Most activities and treatments that help with depression can also help manage anxiety.

There are three concepts related to anxiety that are somewhat unique to the disorder.

Physiological control through deep breathing (i.e., "box breathing") and other recovery practices can be achieved with a little effort and practice. Sometimes referred to as "breath work," this is little more than taking a series of very deep and very slow breaths, holding at the top of the inhale, and exhaling fully. This can help you prepare in advance for a stressful event, calm you if you are already in a state of physiological arousal or panic, and soothe you into a state of deeper consciousness and relaxation. It can also help you fall asleep if you use it in bed at night. I strongly suggest practicing box breathing at least twice a day and whenever you are unable to relax.

Avoidance is the central behavioral aspect of anxiety, and it serves as the primary mechanism that maintains specific forms of anxiety. When we fear something, we try to avoid it. This works really well in many potentially dangerous situations that sensibly require avoidance. For example, I am unwilling to walk down a dark alley in a strange city by myself, so I will walk a few blocks out of my way to avoid it. In modern life, however, behavioral avoidance can come at a high cost relative to the actual risk. One of the most common fears shared by people is the dread of public speaking, even though we can rationally understand that standing in front of a room to tell a story is almost never a dangerous activity.

During my college years, I felt so anxious about public speaking that I would drop a course at the beginning of the semester if class presentations were a requirement. But guess what? Because I successfully avoided college presentations, I never got over my anxiety. During my second year in graduate school, I was assigned to teach an undergraduate course with 350 students. Yikes! I either had to suck it up and teach the course, or my new psychology career would suffer. (Obviously, I sucked it up. By the end of the semester, I became more comfortable standing at the lectern.)

Habituation is one of the simplest forms of learning. It is a change in response to a stimulus after repeated or constant exposure. This involves both psychological and biological processes. A simple example: If you turn on a ceiling fan you will hear it whirring. But sit beneath it for a while and soon you will stop "hearing" it, or at least stop registering the sound between your ears and your brain. If it shuts off, however, you will immediately hear the difference, noticing the change in sound. This is an example of perceptual habituation. Learning that the fan noise is irrelevant, allows you to allocate your attention elsewhere.

The military uses a variation of habituation to prepare soldiers for combat. Think about your military training and how intense it was. Yes, you were honing skills and tactics, but you were also being repetitively exposed to aspects of the dangerous environment you were preparing for. Through training, you learned to be less physiologically reactive before and after actual combat than those without that training. I've heard many operators attribute much of their success to being "calm," "comfortable," or "cool," while the bad guys were panicking.

In treating anxiety disorders, exposure-based psychotherapies are the most effective therapies. The goal of these therapies is to use the principle of habituation to help the patient "learn" not to respond with the physiological arousal associated with anxiety. Returning to my own example, why did I gradually become less anxious teaching that class over the course of a semester? At the start of the very first class, I was sweating, hyperventilating, and my heart was racing. Classic "flight or fight" response involving the sympathetic nervous system. But the longer I stood at the lectern talking—both within classes and across classes—that physiological response gradually modified. My mind and body as a system had habituated to the situation. It "learned" that public speaking was actually not a threatening activity. (If you are one of the many who are anxious about delivering a presentation to others, you can pay a psychotherapist to treat you—or you can join Toastmasters and get the "treatment" for free.)

Some Things You Can Do Now

Review your risk history. Do you have a family history of anxiety? Have you ever been diagnosed with or treated for PTSD or an anxiety disorder?

Evaluate your current status. Are you currently feeling anxious? How many of the symptoms above do you have and how severe are they? Do people who know you well think you are anxious? Do you avoid any situations, activities, or people because they might make you anxious?

Consider lifestyle factors. Is there anything (e.g., animal, situation, place, thing) you consistently avoid because it would cause you anxiety? Is anxiety interfering with your ability to function, sleep, perform your job, or enjoy leisure time? Do you practice good sleep hygiene? Do you have regular social contact with people you care for and trust? Do you use drugs or alcohol to self-medicate?

Decide if you need professional treatment. If you have chronic or severe symptoms of anxiety, you should probably consider seeking treatment.

Final Thoughts on Anxiety

Anxiety can overwhelm functioning, general health, and quality of life, but it is also treatable. If you are highly anxious, ask for, seek out, and find the therapeutics that will help you. They are out there. If one treatment doesn't work for you, try something new: book a float tank session at a local spa, download a meditation app, read up on stellate ganglion block treatment, take up jiujitsu, or simply reorganize your daily schedule to ensure that you have some quiet personal time in the morning and in the evening.

CHAPTER 8

ANGER

"I thought being angry and depressed was just part of being a normal civilian."
—**Patrick Jones**, U.S. Navy, Naval Special Warfare, intelligence analyst

"I learned he spent years training with the knowledge that any mistake could result in death, meaning errors of any size were unacceptable. This helped me to empathize with his source of anger and reassure him during times of potential 'crisis,' like when a lid may be left off a container."
—**Corrie Burton**, U.S. Army Special Forces fiancée

"Once every few months, I have a day where I show up to work and imagine throwing my computer through a window. Usually, I can feel the rage coming, and so I'll reschedule meetings so that I can go on a long ruck or just get out of the office and into nature. It sucks, because I usually don't feel them coming until the morning of."
—**Pete McGuyer**, U.S. Marine Chief Petty Officer, Reconnaissance and Marine Special Operations Command

A few years ago, I received an SOS request to speak with an operator who was living in a hotel, separated from his family. Two nights before, during a drunken argument with his wife, he prevented her from leaving with their children by shooting out a couple tires on her car. He did this in front of his family and neighbors. *Not good.*

How many situations like this have you heard about?

I have heard of guys kicking TVs, throwing drinks, punching themselves in the face (a self-administered black eye!), taking a hammer to a motorcycle, cursing their own children, chasing down other vehicles that cut them off, burning letters and mementos, driving across country just to get away, primal screaming, shooting holes in a wall, and many other things—including direct physical violence.

Marriages have been destroyed, jobs lost, lives upended.

––––––––

It is a widely accepted article of faith that combat veterans are likely to have anger "issues," and many do, but what does that even mean and what are the causes and solutions?

Anger is a human emotion—one of the basic human emotions, meaning it is universal, found in every culture around the world. Other basic emotions include happiness, sadness, anxiety, surprise, and disgust. All these emotions, including anger, are survival mechanisms that have evolved in our ancestors over tens of thousands of years.

Anger is related to the "fight or flight" response. It prepares and motivates us to fight or resist, which is often necessary in life. It does this by triggering an internal state of discomfort, uncertainty, and activation.

As a basic human emotion, anger has a number of universal physiological and behavioral features. An angry facial expression is easily read by most people the world over, featuring frowning, facial tensing, and flushing. In addition, muscles tense up in the neck, shoulders, arms, etc.

Anger affects reason and cognitive functioning. It impairs analytical thinking and judgment, and it erodes trust in others.

Common angry behaviors include yelling, cursing, talking loudly, gesturing with hands, stomping feet, threatening, throwing things, breaking or damaging things, fighting—even suicide. Obviously, these behaviors can lead to trouble—physical injuries, broken property, damaged relationships, and criminal charges.

Risk factors for anger management problems include XY chromosomes, sleep deprivation, chronic pain, depression, anxiety, PTSD, low testosterone, TBI, prior history of violence, family history of violence, addiction, significant loss and grief, betrayal, and more.

Sound familiar?

All military special operators, by virtue of their profession, have a "prior history of violence," including years of lethal training and combat. They are comfortable with firearms and violence. They have been taught to use violence to solve certain types of problems. Rage and violence may even be seen as central to survival. (Remember, anger does have an evolutionary basis, a protective purpose.)

Commonly, operators may direct their anger inward so as not to elicit a violent or scared reaction from others. That is fine, up to a point. But holding anger inside can cause problems too. It's not good for us, especially our cardiac system and our psyche. Feeling chronically angry, especially in social isolation, is absolutely miserable.

It might be a good idea to avoid specific situations where conflict is probable or to withdraw from situations after conflict develops. However, that's not always possible, or even necessarily desirable. The old cliché about "counting to ten" before responding, is actually pretty decent advice if you can make it work. But counting to ten may not be enough—sometimes we have to count to a hundred or more. The best way to do that is to withdraw from a situation—at least temporarily.

Creating a quiet space for some period of time can be helpful. Use box breathing, meditation, music, or physical exercise to calm yourself, reappraise the situation, and plan out the most appropriate response you can make. Then reengage. Solve the problem. Have the conversation. Once you have done everything you can do, let it go. If anger is a problem in your relationships with others, you may need to develop "ground rules" for how you handle conflict. Such rules commonly include "advance directives," such as a specified cooling-off period.

There are many solutions to immediate anger management problems: sleep, relaxation and recovery practices, counting to ten, cognitive reappraisal of situations, among others. More broadly, anything that addresses the other conditions in this book will indirectly reduce anger-related problems.

Cognitive behavioral therapy, anger management, and problem-solving can all help address anger problems directly. Anger management skills can be learned. Counseling can also provide an opportunity to talk about feelings, frustrations, and relationship difficulties, including couples therapy, which can improve communication and conflict resolution between you and your partner.

Some Things You Can Do Now

Review your risk history. Over the past few years, how often have you lost control of your anger and behaved in a way that you later regretted? Do you have a history of tantrums or violence? Have you ever been injured in or arrested for a physical altercation? Has your anger ever damaged an important relationship with someone else?

Evaluate your current status. How often are you angry? How do you behave when you are angry? Does anger currently effect your important relationships?

Decide if you need professional treatment. If you think you need help with your anger, then you probably do.

Final Thoughts on Anger

Anger is a miserable emotion to feel, and it can potentially destroy every single thing you care about. It is commonly associated with most of the conditions within Operator Syndrome. Fortunately, anything that helps treat insomnia, low T, depression, chronic pain, addiction, and other syndrome conditions will also help reduce anger and improve anger management. In particular, it may be helpful to enlist a spouse or someone you confide in for a discussion on how you *actually* handle your anger versus how you would *prefer* to handle your anger.

CHAPTER 9

HYPERVIGILANCE

"Situational awareness."

—**Sun Tzu** (roughly translated)

"Heads on a swivel."

—**Unknown**

"Got your six."

—**Unknown World War I fighter pilot**

"When I left the SEAL teams, it was after multiple deployments to Iraq and Afghanistan. I didn't realize it at first, but working in NYC, riding the subways, constantly being surrounded by millions of people, I was always hypervigilant. I was always scanning the surroundings looking for threats. I realized every time I rode the subway, I would put my back in the corner and constantly survey the passengers looking for anything out of the ordinary. From the second I went into the city until I got home into my bed, I was

on high alert, ready for the next attack. I inevitably broke down, as our bodies can't maintain this state."

—**Jonathan D. Wilson**, former U.S. Navy SEAL, cofounder and former CEO SEAL Future Foundation

Hypervigilance is an official symptom of post-traumatic stress disorder. It appears in PTSD questionnaires and diagnostic interviews. Mental health clinicians often regard it as though it is just another symptom that must be "treated." But it is more than just a "symptom"—much more—because it is also an effective behavioral adaptation. Focused vigilance is what keeps soldiers alive in unpredictable and dangerous environments. Over time, it soon develops into a reflex, a survival instinct that is hard to override, even at home.

And this makes sense: The habits that keep us alive become deeply engrained. They endure. We do not want to let go of them. They become part of our identity. Some common examples of hypervigilance include the following:

- Feeling on "high alert"
- Being "keyed up" about personal security concerns
- Tracking all potential exits in a restaurant
- Safety positioning
- Scrutinizing and watching everyone who comes and goes
- Running scenarios in your mind
- Watching and memorizing vehicles behind you while driving
- Evasive driving, changing lanes under bypasses, avoiding manholes and road debris

- Aggressive driving to avoid traffic jams, choke points, or anyone who has followed you for more than two turns
- Carrying a concealed weapon away from home
- Frequently checking windows and doors at home
- "Zoning out" while your spouse is talking because your mind is focused on security issues
- Listening for sounds while in bed
- Investigating the slightest unusual noise
- Tactically clearing the house in the middle of the night with a firearm

Sound familiar?

There is a downside to hypervigilance. What kept an operator alive in perilous environments may not be as necessary at home. And it comes at a cost—a cost to the operator and a cost to the family.

Maintaining a constant state of "high alert" means that one is in a chronic state of overactivation of the sympathetic nervous system. It means a constant physiological surge of cortisol and other stress chemicals, which adversely affects us in many ways, including insomnia, depression, hormonal disruption, and anxiety.

Extreme hypervigilance can mean not being present in the moment with one's family. It can lead to exhaustion, an inability to relax or enjoy time with family, insomnia, irritation of a spouse, and long-term harmful effects to brain and body. Often social withdrawal and avoidance of the outside world are downstream effects of hypervigilance. If your home is a secure "compound," you may be reluctant to ever leave it.

This is not to say there is zero risk of danger in most developed countries, but the threat environment in Smalltown

U.S.A. is obviously very different than it is in Kandahar or Ramadi. Your vigilance behaviors may not be commensurate to the actual danger in your environment.

There are cognitive and behavioral ways to seek a balance of vigilance. Implement sensible environmental engineering at home. Harden the target. Use good locks, redundant alarm systems, dogs that will bark, and self-defense weapons. Concealed carry may also be your friend. I support that.

Take reasonable precautions—absolutely—but don't limit yourself to installed security measures. There is more you can do.

Try a little cognitive therapy on yourself to see if there are ways you can help yourself relax more and engage with your family. Maybe this would be a good moment to reflect on the "Serenity Prayer":

> God, grant me the serenity to accept the things
> I cannot change,
> Courage to change the things I can,
> And wisdom to know the difference.

It might be helpful to have a discussion with your spouse. Your buddies might also have ideas.

Analyze the threat risk in your usual environment. Conduct an appraisal of the threats in your world, your home, and the places you want to go to, including the places your family wants you to go to.

How actually dangerous is it in your neighborhood? What are the types of potential threats? How likely are they? And if you have practical security and defense measures in place, how comfortable can you allow yourself to be at home?

What are the risks to you personally of going out to a store, a restaurant, or a theater? How do those risks evolve if your family is with you? What reasonable steps can you plan in advance so that these risks are mitigated sufficiently?

One way to evaluate the probability of a risk is to compare it to that of other *known* risks. Driving is a good example to use. For example, we know how many Americans die in motor vehicle accidents every year (about forty-three thousand in 2021, which are the highest total fatalities since 2007). And we know about how many miles Americans drive in a year. The ratio of fatalities per one hundred million people times the total vehicle miles traveled between 2020 and 2021 was 1.3, the highest ratio since 2007 (but far better than historical averages before 2007).

So, there is risk to driving. National statistics show that people die, at the rate of forty-three thousand per year. Every time we get behind the wheel, we face the very real possibility of being in a severe or fatal accident.

And that's why we, as a society, take the best precautions we can. We have driver regulations, seatbelts, airbags, driver-assist, regular vehicle maintenance, stop signs and stoplights, and so on. We mitigate risk as best we reasonably can… *and then we keep on driving.* Why? Because collectively we accept the risk, given that using trucks or cars has considerable benefits. In fact, our risk-*benefit* analysis tells us it's okay to keep driving, so long as we are careful, follow rules, and use protective technology.

Now consider which is more dangerous: sitting in a restaurant or driving to that restaurant? I don't have a data-driven, actuarial answer to that question right now, but give it some thought. What is the best balance of vigilance and relaxation?

What ground rules and principles can you construct for your-self? Maybe there are reasonable measures to take, planned in advance, that will allow you to relax and be present for your family—and yourself.

CHAPTER 10

PTSD

"War in itself is not as traumatic as is presumed. It is particular personal losses that haunt me, especially where I believe I should have done something different beforehand."

—**Mark Ozdarski**, U.S. Navy SEAL (Ret.)

"PTSD is a syndrome-based classification system that adheres to the DSM's 'assumption of healthy normality,' thereby rendering any behavior deviating from 'normal' as pathological. What does this assumption of healthy normality mean for our SOF operators? Is it even relevant to them? Their profession demands distinct behavioral adaptations for survival in combat environments—contexts where pain is a natural consequence of the human experience and a destructive normality is presumed."

—**Michael Vollmer**, PsyD, U.S. Navy Lieutenant, Military Sealift Command and SEAL, licensed clinical psychologist

*"The biggest disservice we do to our operators is subject them to the normal healthcare system, where providers tell them that **nothing***

*is wrong with them—or that it's **PTSD**. We should provide our operators with appropriate job- and risk-specific care."*
—**Dr. Jennifer Byrne**, U.S. Air Force veteran, U.S. Air Force Pararescueman spouse

Post-traumatic stress disorder (PTSD) is one of the most common psychiatric disorders among veterans. It is a relatively new diagnosis, first established in 1980. This means we only have forty-plus years of research to guide our understanding of how to understand, diagnose, and treat this condition.

To be diagnosed with PTSD, one must have experienced something traumatic, such as a physical or sexual assault, motor vehicle accident, a close brush with death in a natural disaster, or combat experiences. There are four categories of symptoms with this disorder:

1. Reexperiencing the trauma in some form, such as flashbacks, nightmares, frightening thoughts, or strong emotional or physiological reactions to being reminded of the traumatic event. The central feature of these symptoms is fear reactivity; that is, reacting with a "fight or flight" response when reexperiencing traumatic memories or cues.

2. Avoidance of traumatic memories and reminders. This includes avoidance of thoughts or feelings related to the traumatic event. It also includes avoidance of people, places, or activities that might be reminders of the traumatic event. The aim of its sufferer is to avoid anything that will provoke fear reactivity. As with all other

anxiety disorders, avoidance behaviors inadvertently serve to maintain the symptoms of anxiety and distress.

3. Arousal symptoms, including hypervigilance, exaggerated startle reactions, sleep disturbance, and anger. These arousal symptoms overlap with mood and anxiety disorders, as well as other conditions, and are therefore not necessarily unique to PTSD.

4. Symptoms of mood and thoughts that are highly negative, such as self-blame, guilt, loss of activities previously enjoyed, sadness, loss of pleasure and joy in life, and social isolation. These mood symptoms overlap with mood and anxiety disorders and are not unique to PTSD.

As you may have noticed, PTSD has become the go-to psychosocial diagnosis for the VA system. It seems that any veteran who was previously deployed to a war zone is likely to be diagnosed with PTSD if they report any form of psychological difficulty or interpersonal problem. Not only does the VA fund the largest mental health system in the world, but they also provide lifetime cash disability benefits for veterans diagnosed with PTSD.

So far, over half of all veterans who served in the Global War on Terror since 9/11 have already applied for VA disability benefits for PTSD. That's over 50 percent, even though rigorous epidemiological studies suggest the actual rate of combat PTSD is only about 8 percent, and a majority of those cases are mild or moderate in severity. As you might expect, whenever you provide a significant financial incentive for a behavior, such as reporting symptoms of PTSD, you are certain to see more of that behavior. Moreover, the VA is unable to show *any* administrative evidence of treatment effectiveness for the billions of dollars they spend on mental health treatment programs for veterans. As an old axiom in medicine states: "It is hard to get better when you have to prove you are sick."

———

So, what is PTSD, really?

Here is how I view PTSD: I see it as a combination of depression and anxiety symptoms, plus fear reactivity, that is specific to the nature of the trauma experienced. Fear reactivity and associated avoidance is the core feature of PTSD. You can be a combat veteran with symptoms of depression and anxiety, but unless you have intrusive memories and experiences of fear reactivity to past traumas, you do not have PTSD as it is actually defined by American psychiatry. Expressed as a formula, it can look like this:

PTSD = depression + anxiety + fear reactivity with possible avoidance

One implication of this conceptualization of PTSD is that it may not be an actual specific and unique disorder, but rather a combination of other psychiatric disorders that develop from a trauma-specific context—and have trauma-specific manifestations such as nightmares or feeling distress when confronted with reminders. Perhaps what we call "PTSD" is a mixture of depression and anxiety within the context of personal tragedy.

There is another perspective on PTSD from the medical field of neurology. In a landmark paper published in 2012, Sharon Shively and Daniel Perl, two neurological pathologists at the Uniformed Services University of the Health Sciences, reviewed the history of how we came to understand and label TBI and PTSD as seen in combatants.

What was called "shell shock" during World War I was thought at the time to be a neurological condition caused by the unrelenting, high-energy explosive artillery fire of trench warfare in France. However, over two decades after the war, this neurological perspective lost out to the burgeoning discipline of psychiatry, and the influential theories of Sigmund Freud and Carl Jung. "Shell shock," conceived of as a neurological injury to the brain, gave way to psychodynamic theories—including untested notions of the unconscious mind—that have shaped the field of psychiatry since its inception.

For these and other reasons, there are now voices calling to change how we identify the phenomenon known as PTSD, converting it from a "disorder" to an "injury"—in other words, post-traumatic stress injury, or PTSI, rather than PTSD.

———

In my work with the special operations community, I have found relatively little evidence of PTSD in its prototypical form—that is, with fear reactivity and avoidance as central symptoms. Most operators deny that they experience crippling fear or avoidance reactions related to thoughts or cues associated with their military experiences. In fact, many say they enjoyed their combat deployments and would do it all over again if they could.

But if you do have PTSD, I want you to know that, like depression and anxiety disorders, PTSD is a highly treatable condition.

It is not a life sentence!

The VA might have you believe otherwise, and as a system, it has never publicly shown any administrative data on the effectiveness of their PTSD treatment programs. This strongly suggests that veterans are not getting better with the treatment the VA provides. In contrast, civilians treated for PTSD generally get much better, and many reach a point of full recovery. In fact, even without any treatment, about half of all civilians with PTSD will recover naturally over time.

While you may think that combat trauma is unique from other forms of trauma, past research shows that symptoms and personality testing profiles for combat veterans and sexual assault survivors are virtually identical prior to treatment.

From a psychiatric treatment perspective, interventions for PTSD are essentially the same as for depression and anxiety disorders. The interventions I described earlier in Chapters 6 and 7 are the same ones we use for PTSD. Psychotherapy and antidepressant medications are usually tried first. The psychotherapy is likely to have specific adaptations related to the nature of the traumas, including some form of exposure to traumatic memories. Usually this involves talking or writing about past traumas.

In recent years, novel therapies have shown powerful benefits for treating the constellation of symptoms commonly associated with PTSD in military special operators. These include stellate ganglion block therapy, which directly targets the sympathetic nervous system (a.k.a. the "fight or flight" system), ketamine infusions, magnetic electroencephalogram resonance therapy (MeRT), and psychedelic medicines such as ibogaine and 5-MeO-DMT. These interventions are described and discussed in Chapter 21.

Further Recommended Readings

- "Traumatic Brain Injury, Shell Shock, and Posttraumatic Stress Disorder in the Military—Past, Present, and Future" by Sharon Shively and Daniel Perl in the *Journal of Head Trauma and Rehabilitation* 27 (2012): 234–239
- "Why Are Iraq and Afghanistan War Veterans Seeking PTSD Disability Compensation at Unprecedented Rates?" by Richard McNally and Christopher Frueh in the *Journal of Anxiety Disorder* 27 (2013): 520–526
- *The End of Trauma: How the New Science of Resilience is Changing How We Think About PTSD* by George Bonanno, PhD (Basic Books, 2021)
- *The Invisible Machine: The Startling Truth About Trauma and the Scientific Breakthrough That Can Transform Your Life* by Eugene Lipov, MD and Jamie Mustard (BenBella Books, 2023)

CHAPTER 11

SUBSTANCE ABUSE

"Drinking was a part of the culture I had been a part of my entire adult life. I never did it in moderation. I used alcohol and other substances to minimize anxiety and aggression and depression. Sobriety allowed me to see the problems clearly, address them the way they deserved, and save myself and my marriage before I allowed it to spiral out of control. I had to be sober-minded and go through the process and deal with the residual of the bad times."
—**Chad White**, U.S. Army Special Forces Sergeant
First Class (Ret.)

"The evolution from daily drinking to excessive drinking to being a blackout drunk took time to develop, but I never understood why. I felt alone, thrown away, and filled with regret. When my family was taken from me because of my actions, I was in a personal hell. The lowest of lows. Rock bottom. I was in a state of ending everything when a friend put me in touch with someone who might help. I was given the Operator Syndrome paper and that literally saved my life. I read it over and over, studied it, highlighted all the parts that pertained to me, and I felt understood.

I realized I was not alone. I wasn't the only one experiencing so many symptoms. It helped my family understand my situation. It started my journey towards recovery and understanding. It was the turning point I desperately needed."

—**Dave Gibbons**, U.S. Army Special Forces (Ret.)

When you don't really care so much whether you live or die, it's easy to take another drink. It's also easy to take another drink when you're feeling stressed out, struggling with pain, anxious, angry, depressed, or lonely. Alcohol and other drugs are often used to help people cope, relax, enjoy social activities, and sleep. This is often described as "self-medicating."

Drinking is culturally normative in most, if not all, SOF units. Often it is virtually a competitive sport, and the peer pressure to imbibe can be tremendous. The other guys might not trust you if you don't drink with them. Use of other mind-altering or performance-enhancing substances is also common, including nicotine, steroids, and painkillers (which are widely prescribed).

It is understandable that someone who is suffering would look for relief. To "self-medicate" is perfectly understandable, and it is common among operators. However, alcohol and drugs can cause both acute and chronic problems, furthering the damage caused by TBI, insomnia, depression, and anxiety.

Alcohol is a depressant, and it fragments sleep. So, while it may seem to help you fall asleep, it is really only causing you to pass out. Most people who have more than three drinks in the evening are likely to wake up several times throughout the night, which interrupts the natural sleep cycle, which, in turn, leads to disruptions in REM and slow-wave deep sleep. This is terrible for an already-injured brain. Over time, chronic heavy alcohol use is also depressing your central nervous system, making depression worse.

When I ask guys how many alcoholic drinks they typically have, I know there are important follow-up questions that also have to be asked. If a guy tells me he usually has two drinks a day, I have to inquire what form of alcohol he drinks and how large each drink is. I've had guys tell me with a straight face that they only have two cocktails a night—and then on follow-up, I learn their definition of "one cocktail" is to take an eighteen-ounce glass, add a few ice cubes, a splash of cranberry, and then fill it to the rim from a handle of vodka.

Most people know that the current medical thinking on alcohol is that men should not have more than two drinks a day, and women should not have more than one drink. Heavier drinking on a regular basis can cause liver disease, heart disease, cancer, weight gain, and brain damage (e.g., Korsakoff syndrome).

These medical recommendations are based on what is known as a "standard drink size," which allows for setting equivalencies between different types of alcohol. One domestic beer (about 5 percent alcohol) is one standard drink; for higher octane IPAs that may be 6 percent, 9 percent, or higher in alcohol content, one must recalculate accordingly. Equivalent to this one domestic beer is one glass of wine (four to five ounces) or 1.5 ounces of spirits (at 40 percent alcohol or 80 proof), or written more simply:

1 "Standard Drink" = 1 beer = 1 glass of wine = 1.5 ounces of spirits (80 proof)

An ounce and a half of alcohol is actually not as much as most people think. Remember the "three martini lunches" of the good old days? Prior to the 1970s it used to be that a typical martini served in a bar or restaurant was made with one ounce of gin or vodka. If you ever watch any of the old black and white *Thin Man* movies, you'll notice that while William Powell always seems to have a martini in his hand, the size of the glass is barely larger than a thimble! We have supersized many things in America, including our cocktails. Nowadays it is not unusual to receive three to five ounces of liquor when we order a martini—the equivalent of two or three standard drinks!

Binge drinking of alcohol is defined as having five or more standard sized drinks on one occasion for a man, or four or more drinks for a woman. This is very dangerous, and can lead to alcohol poisoning, interpersonal violence, legal trouble, and serious accidents. (My own father died during a binge-drinking episode when he fell down a flight of stairs and received a massive brain injury. His blood alcohol at the time of death was almost three times the legal blood-alcohol limit for driving.)

Heavy drinking on a chronic basis is also a major risk to health and relationships, and it leaves one vulnerable to all kinds of other trouble. Addiction overall involves a two-factor biological process (tolerance and withdrawal), as well as physiological and behavioral conditioning, detailed below:

- **Tolerance.** When we drink alcohol (or use most any other drug) on a daily or regular basis, we gradually begin to need more of the juice in order to get the same high. Thus, one drink a night becomes two, then three, etc. At this point, it's very difficult to cut back on the stuff, because to do so, even a little, generally means discomfort. To quit "cold turkey," or cut back substantially all at once, likely means some level of withdrawal sickness.

- **Withdrawal.** If we abruptly stop drinking or using after we've developed a tolerance, we are likely to get sick. Withdrawal usually involves, at minimum, increased anxiety, depression, and irritability. It can also mean cold sweats, tremors, nausea, and vomiting. At the severe end of the spectrum, it can lead to seizures or even heart attacks. Usually, we would advise someone with a heavy use habit to cut down gradually (easier said than done) or seek medical help with alcohol detox. This usually involves spending a few days on a detox unit, receiving fluids and benzodiazepines (e.g., Valium) to help the body get past the withdrawal stage without getting too sick or risking a cardiovascular event.

- **Conditioning.** Most addictions also involve some degree of physiological and behavioral conditioning. Our bodies and our psyche are accustomed to our habit, and we are likely to miss it at times—even after the withdrawal period is well over. This is the reason people are encouraged to change up some of their routines. Don't drive past that bar where you did a lot of your drinking. Don't hang out with friends who are drinking. Certain foods, social activities, and even moods that have been associated with the substance use are likely to cue up cravings and the risk of relapse.

For these and other reasons, addictions are extremely difficult to get over. Adding to the challenges of tolerance, withdrawal, and conditioning is the reality that if the substance of choice has been used as a form of self-medication, its sudden absence is especially difficult to manage, and replacement strategies will be important to cultivate.

While alcohol is probably the most commonly abused mind-altering substance, use and abuse of other substances is also common, including nicotine, cannabis, and opiates.

Many guys use nicotine to help sooth anxiety and improve focus. In and of itself, nicotine may not pose a health risk. However, smoking cigarettes or "dipping" tobacco is obviously a carcinogen. Smoking anything is not good for our lungs. Using nicotine patches or gum is a healthier delivery method, but it can also lead to increased use and tolerance due to the ease of delivery.

Cannabis is used by many to help with relaxation, sleep, nausea, and pain management. Obviously, edibles (e.g., gummies or chocolates), oils, or tinctures are much healthier alternatives to smoking it. Even though it is available medically or recreationally in many states, be mindful that the medical benefits of cannabis have not really been well-studied. Cannabis does not have a traditional addiction profile for most people who use it, but sudden withdrawal after regular use may still lead to a period of increased anxiety and irritability.

Opiates are widely prescribed for acute and chronic pain, and they have clear implications for addiction, abuse, and overdose. We build up tolerance to opiates very quickly, within a matter of days, and the withdrawal affects are especially nasty. Moreover, the risk of a fatal overdose, especially when used concurrently with alcohol or other drugs is high. In 2021, there were over 106,000 fatal overdoses in the U.S., driven to a large extent by illegal fentanyl, a fivefold increase from 2000 when there were fewer than twenty thousand overdose deaths.

There are several different approaches to moderating or ending an addiction. Some people do it themselves without any help, while others rely on medical treatment or peer-support programs, such as Alcoholics Anonymous. Here are some options:

- **Detoxification.** A medical detox is often advisable for severe alcohol, opiate, or stimulant (e.g., meth) addictions. This usually involves spending three to seven days on a detox ward—or it may be completed at home with medical advice, prescription detox medications, and strong social support.

- **Abstinence models.** The intended goal of abstinence models is exactly that: complete abstinence—not one taste of the juice, ever. Treatment success is measured in days, weeks, months, and years of continuous abstinence. Any relapse at all, no matter how small, resets the clock or calendar back to the beginning. Alcoholics Anonymous and other twelve-step community programs follow this approach.

- **Harm reduction.** This is an approach to managing addiction that does not set abstinence as the only definition of success. It takes the perspective that reductions in harmful use are also worthwhile. If a heavy drinker can cut back from a bottle of bourbon a day to a half-bottle a day, that is a significant reduction in harm. It's still not truly healthy, but it represents a significant improvement, and one that abstinence models don't recognize. It also allows people with addiction to reduce their use in small increments, with each increment representing a "win" without the pressure to achieve an outcome of perfection all at once (i.e., full abstinence).

- **Inpatient or residential sobriety programs.** Inpatient treatment, commonly twenty-eight-day programs, typically involves staying in a locked hospital ward. These programs of confinement usually include medical detox, as well as individual and group therapies, with a lot of education and restructuring of habits and coping skills. Residential sobriety programs, on the other hand, are places to live while developing the structure and habits of sobriety. Such programs are generally not hospital-based and usually allow for outside work or visitation.

- **Medications.** Several medications have shown moderate effectiveness at helping to manage alcohol and opiate abuse, especially when used in combination with counseling. Naltrexone (not to be confused with naloxone, which is used to reverse an opioid overdose) is a prescription medication that helps to reduce substance use cravings, and it mostly eliminates the "high" from alcohol and opiates. It is an opioid antagonist, which means it works by blocking opioid receptors throughout the central nervous system. In addition to naltrexone, there are other medications that act similarly, such as acamprosate. These medications don't make you sick if you drink or use, but if you don't get the euphoric buzz from that bottle of bourbon, you're much more likely to stop drinking from it. (A person who is still opioid-dependent should not use naltrexone until after they have detoxed.)

What medical or community treatment approaches show the most effectiveness? There is no clear winner; all approaches seem to have about the same rate of efficacy, and we cannot as yet predict which approach will be most effective for any given individual.

About one third of the those who attempt any form of addiction intervention will achieve success—and two thirds won't. The odds are not great for any single substance abuse treatment effort. Relapse—after some period of full sobriety or reduced harm—is the most common outcome.

Do not let that deter you.

A few weeks of sobriety is nonetheless a meaningful form of harm reduction. It gives your liver and other organs a chance to heal themselves, at least partially. It also allows you to see what life is like when you are not using heavily. You are likely to see realities that you hadn't previously noticed, such as the effect your drinking has had on your partner or family.

We also know that even when there is a relapse after substance abuse treatment efforts, lessons are still learned. Failure is one of our best teachers. We learn what worked and what didn't, and we develop a better awareness of the cues, environments, and emotions that trigger a relapse. Best of all? That one-third chance of success is still there the next time we make a serious effort at curbing our addiction. Persistence pays off. Given the law of averages, with three or four attempts, most people will achieve a healthier balance of their substance use.

Some Things You Can Do Now

Review your risk history. Do you have a past history of heavy alcohol or drug use? Have you ever been diagnosed with or treated for an addiction? Did either of your parents or grand-parents have a substance use problem?

Evaluate your current status. How often do you drink or use? How many standard-sized alcoholic drinks do you typically have at one time when you drink? How often do you have five or more drinks on one occasion? Has any friend or loved one told you that you have a substance use problem recently? Has your substance use caused you any problems recently, such as legal trouble, violence or conflict at home, accidents, or trouble with employment?

Consider lifestyle factors. Do you often use alcohol or drugs to make it through a day or a night? Do you use alcohol or drugs to cope with any particular situations, stressors, or subjective internal experiences (e.g., depression, pain)?

Decide if you need professional treatment. Be honest with yourself. If you think you might have a problem, discuss the issue with someone you trust, make a plan, and execute.

Final Thoughts on Substance Abuse

Alcohol and drugs have devastated the lives of many operators and their families. This devastation can be slow and gradual, or sudden and acute. Alcohol and drugs are implicated in many, many instances of domestic violence and suicide. Please take corrective action if you need to.

CHAPTER 12

PERCEPTUAL SYSTEM IMPAIRMENTS

Sensation and perception together are a subdiscipline of the field of psychology (often known as "S and P") and every introductory textbook to psychology includes a chapter on it. I have no specialty training in vision care, audiology, or kinesiology, but I know just enough to be dangerous.

Let's start with a brief conceptual foundation. We experience the outside world around us via our senses of vision, hearing, smell, taste, touch, and proprioception (our sense of self-movement and position). Each of our perceptual systems include biological versions of "hardware" that gather data and "software" that manages and analyzes that data. These systems provide us with information critical to our ability to function—information that we experience psychologically, or in our mind.

Sensation occurs when a sensory organ (eyes, ears, nose, mouth, skin, or the vestibular system located in the inner ear) receives physical stimuli from the universe and converts it into patterns of nervous system signals that are sent to specialized processing centers in our brain.

Our eyes, for example, are a very complex and delicate instrument (i.e., "hardware") that receive light energy (typically four hundred to seven hundred nanometers on the electromagnetic spectrum). Light waves are received through an opening in the eyeball (i.e., the pupil), focused through a lens (which is adjusted to be thicker or thinner by tiny ciliary muscles), passed through the vitreous humor (the jelly-like substance inside our eyeball), and brought to the retina at the back of our eyeball. The retina is a layer of photoreceptors (i.e., rods and cones), which convert the light-formed images into nervous system signals that are then transmitted down the optic nerve to the specialized vision processing center at the back of our brain.

Perception is the processing and interpretation of those signals by these specialized centers in our brain. Each of our senses has its own specialized processing area or areas in the brain.

Sensation and perception represent two parts of a process that allows us to experience the world around us. In other words, "hardware" collects the raw data, and "software" interprets that data and sends out messages to the relevant parts of our central nervous system. Both sensation and perception are necessary to for us to see, hear, smell, touch, taste, and maintain balance.

If we damage the sensory hardware (e.g., our eyes), then there are no signals to send to be processed in the brain. If we damage the specialized area of our brain that interprets sensory signals, then we will impair or eliminate our ability to interpret—or make sense of—the signals. We can also damage the "wiring" that connects our sensory organs to the brain.

Each of our senses may be blocked or impaired by problems at any point along this process. For example, the hardware of our eyeballs can be injured or diseased. Poke the surface of the eye with a stick, and it may be damaged and unable to collect light energy. Further along, if we expose the delicate ciliary muscles to blast waves, the lens may lose its ability to focus well. At the end of the process, a blow to the head can damage the software of our brain's visual processing center.

Our perceptions do not reproduce reality. Even under the best of conditions, we can be tricked into misinterpreting the incoming data. Accurate perception involves learning and context. Hand-eye coordination, for example, must be learned at specific critical periods during an animal's development; if that period is missed, there is very little chance to catch up. Young kittens fitted with a cone that prevents them from seeing their paws for several weeks will later have great difficulty coordinating their paws and vision after the cone is removed.

Optical illusions are another example of perceptual fallibility. A full moon looks bigger when it hovers just above the horizon than when it is overhead, even though we know the size or proximity of the moon does not change.

———————

Virtually every operator I've known has some level of injury and impairment in at least one of their perceptual systems. The three systems most commonly injured are hearing, vision, and proprioception. Sometimes the sensory organ itself is injured directly, such as an airborne particle impacting an eyeball. Other times, TBIs can affect specialized perception areas in the brain. The following are specific operator injuries and treatments in these perceptual areas:

- **Hearing.** Our ears were neither designed nor have evolved to tolerate exposures to very loud noises. When the intensity or amplitude of sound waves is high, we experience what we perceive as a loud noise. Exposure to gunfire and explosions, acutely or chronically, eventually leads to hearing loss and chronic ringing in the ears (tinnitus). Both hearing loss and tinnitus are common in operators, and both should be evaluated via an audiology exam. Hearing aids are helpful to some with hearing loss, and if they are prescribed or needed, be sure to use them. Set your vanity aside, because there is emerging new research suggesting that untreated hearing loss causes damage to the brain, possibly contributing to dementia later in life. Tinnitus, on the other hand, does not seem to be very treatable. About the best you can do is use white noise to mask the ringing in your ears. A lot of guys run a fan or a sound machine in their bedroom at night.

- **Vision.** Some operators describe having blurry vision, double vision, floaters, trouble seeing at night, or sensitivity to light. Unless there was a direct injury to the eye itself, most of these problems stem from impact forces or blast exposures that affect the visual perception area of the brain. I've also heard of blurry vision thought to be caused by injuries to the delicate ciliary muscles that focus the lens, also probably caused by blast exposures. If you're having any visual problems, go for an optometry or ophthalmology exam. If you're in your early to mid-forties and notice that you have trouble focusing on words and numerals when reading, do not be alarmed by this. It is called presbyopia, and it comes for us all eventually. As we age, our lens loses some of its flexibility and therefore is unable to bring close objects into focus. This is why your parents, grandparents— and at some point, you—require special glasses to read. (You can find these glasses at any drugstore and rarely is an eye exam or prescription needed.)

- **Proprioception or balance.** A classic symptom of TBI is disequilibrium. Many operators report intermittent difficulties with poor balance, dizziness, clumsiness, poor hand-eye coordination, and vertigo symptoms of moving or spinning while still. These symptoms may come and go, may be worse at different times of the day, and might be accompanied by fatigue, nausea, or even vomiting. In my conversations, I frequently hear versions of the following statements:
  - *"I feel unsteady on my feet."*
  - *"Sometimes the room spins."*
  - *"I've become clumsy."*
  - *"I drop things all the time."*
  - *"I no longer feel safe on a ladder."*
  - *"My shoulder is bruised from stumbling into door frames."*
  - *"I don't even trust myself to hold my infant child while standing or walking."*

These symptoms and the functional impairments they cause can be maddening, but they also may be treatable. Vestibular assessment and rehabilitation therapy is a specialty field of physical therapy aimed at reducing difficulties with proprioception. Rehabilitation exercises, repositioning treatments, and balance training can be highly effective and quickly bring great relief. These therapies involve exercises and rehabilitative activities, and they generally do not involve any medications.

CHAPTER 13

COGNITIVE IMPAIRMENTS

"My injuries have most significantly impacted my cognition, memory, light sensitivity, headaches, sleep, and right-eye function. I began doing hyperbaric oxygen therapy (HBOT) in 2015, and since then, I have completed additional dives in 2019 and 2022. The first thing I noticed was the vast improvement with my memory. I was moving to a new area and I was able to remember directions without using my map on my phone to get around. HBOT was not a quick fix for me, but more gradually over time...sleep got better, headaches decreased, light sensitivity has significantly reduced, and my cognition continues improving."

—**Daniel Luna**, EdD, U.S. Navy SEAL (Ret.)

Robert K. was a large man. My estimate put him at six feet three inches, 270 pounds. His muscles stretched and rippled the T-shirt he wore. A wide, sun-burned face and granite jaw gave him an invincible air. He might have come straight from central casting except for one thing: He was sobbing. Tear streaks marked his face.

His career had included two pumps to Iraq with an elite unit of the U.S. Marine Corps, two years in urban law enforcement, and almost eight years of service as a private defense contractor on personal security detail teams, with deployments to Iraq and Afghanistan.

His deployments were notable for heavy urban combat, as well as exposure to frequent indirect fire, vehicle-borne improvised explosive devices (VBIEDs), tactical driving, and ambushes. He had never been medically diagnosed with a concussion, but he estimated he'd had his "bell rung" several dozen times. He had been choked out at least four times in training. He had trained with demolitions and shoulder-fired rockets. He had also been blown up twice by roadway IEDs, losing consciousness both times.

But why exactly was Robert crying? Because his sixteen-year-old son had recently commented on his difficulty holding simple conversations and accused him of being drunk or "messed up" on drugs. The son wanted to move out of his father's house and in with his mother, Robert's ex-wife.

Robert promised me he had been sober for almost a year, and I believed him, but I could see why his son would have thought otherwise. In our conversations, he often had trouble finding words and frequently lost his train of thought mid-sentence. He acknowledged that this had become his "new normal." He described many of the classic cognitive impairments—difficulties with concentration, short-term memory, and organization—that are very common in operators.

Robert's list was a long one, articulated by him as follows:

- I forget about appointments all the time, even with calendar alerts, and that makes people angry.
- I lose my keys and other things around the house.
- I get home from work and realized I'd forgotten something, and I'd have to drive all the way back for it.
- I eventually lost my job because I couldn't keep track of what I was supposed to do.
- I go to the store and then can't remember what I went there to buy.
- I can't recall conversations I have with people, even just a few hours later.
- It takes me longer to complete simple tasks, such as paying the bills, and I make mistakes.
- I can't concentrate to read anything and have to reread passages over two or three times.
- I can't focus even to watch a movie.
- I can't multitask anymore.
- Sometimes while driving, I get lost—even in my own hometown.
- I have trouble completing anything; I have multiple projects going right now.
- I have to check everything I do, multiple times, to be sure I didn't forget and skip a step.
- I can't seem to learn new things, even basic things—learning used to be easy for me.

"I feel so dumb, so incompetent now," Robert concluded. He was no longer crying—just resigned. "Even my own son thinks I'm a drunken fool, and he's lost all respect for me."

Some of the most disruptive symptoms of Operator Syndrome are the cognitive deficits that often develop as a result of TBI, chronic fatigue from insomnia, hormonal dysregulation, and anxiety. These include functional problems with attention, sustained concentration, short- and long-term memory, executive functioning, processing speed, and general intelligence, often measured as IQ. Taken collectively, this also includes trouble staying organized, completing tasks, making decisions, understanding new concepts, learning new material, and remembering things. It is common to have to reread material multiple times or rewatch portions of movies and television shows.

These impairments can be highly distressing and confusing, especially because most operators were highly intelligent problem-solvers during their military career. Cognitive deficits can impair your functioning in many ways and across many situations. They can drive you and the people around you nuts. They are also one of the reasons I strongly encourage operators to enlist the help of a spouse or partner to help them with their healing journey.

Despite these overwhelming difficulties, there is good reason for hope. As you progress through your treatments—as your sleep, hormones, mood, pain, and brain health improve—your cognitive functioning should improve as well.

Several years ago, a retired operator I know enrolled in a comprehensive treatment program for Operator Syndrome. When he began the program, he was extremely depressed and anxious, suffering from insomnia, chronic pain, and TBI. Early in his treatment, a neuropsychologist administered an IQ test and found the operator was performing at about the 84th percentile compared to the general population. A year later and after significant treatment benefits, the same test was administered by the same neuropsychologist. This time the operator's IQ tested out at the 95th percentile, a significant improvement. This was likely a return to his own natural baseline.

This represents a good case use. Neuropsychological performance testing can help to quantify cognitive strengths, weaknesses, and functional deficits related to each of the various areas of cognition. Such testing is not only informative, but also may lead to specific treatment recommendations.

Cognitive behavioral or speech therapies can be very effective for improving cognition. You can also learn what we call compensatory strategies, or adaptations, such as keeping a calendar of meetings and appointments, using a whiteboard at home, compiling notes in a phone or journal, setting up alerts on a mobile phone, and many other simple techniques.

As with most other conditions and functional impairments, there is no simple fix, no magic pill. However, I believe that if you make efforts to steadily address all aspects of Operator Syndrome that are relevant to you, your concentration, memory, and intellectual abilities are likely to improve significantly. In other words: improved sleep, brain health, hormonal health, and emotional health will each lead to improved concentration and memory.

––––––––––

We have addressed many of the effects that TBI can have on the body and psyche, but we haven't talked much about how an injury to the brain affects our thinking. The term "cognitive functioning" is quite broad; it includes attention, sustained concentration, short- and long-term memory, executive functioning, processing speed, and intelligence. TBIs can damage each of these functions individually and collectively. Other aspects of Operator Syndrome can as well. Let's define some of these terms:

- **Attention** is a selective narrowing or focusing of consciousness on a discrete aspect of information. It is the allocation of our very finite cognitive resources to what seems most important at any given moment.
- **Sustained concentration** is the ability to maintain a steady focus of attention on one particular task over the course of time, typically measured in minutes or hours. This is necessary to read a book, cook a meal, complete work tasks, and engage in a meaningful conversation.
- **Memory** involves receiving, storing, retaining, and recalling information. Things can go wrong at any one of those four steps. For example, if you're unable to pay attention to some piece of information, you will not be able to receive or store that information.
- **Information processing speed**, also known as "mental chronometry," is the study of reaction times to complete a range of different cognitive tasks. This cognitive variable is strongly associated with general health and longevity.
- **Executive functioning** requires the simultaneous use of multiple basic cognitive abilities, and includes reasoning, planning, and problem-solving.
- **Intelligence** (often measured as IQ) is a general term that includes each of the prior cognitive domains and

how they work together. Another way to think about intelligence is that it is the combined mental abilities to adapt, shape, and select one's environment. It also includes judgment, comprehension, logical reasoning, and a range of social abilities.

———————

There are practical implications of cognitive impairments. It is more difficult to get along in life if you have difficulties thinking effectively. Not only is it harder for you, but also for those around you. After a TBI, many people find that learning new information is difficult, even though they may retain knowledge and skills they had prior to the TBI. We also know that operators become "task saturated" and overwhelmed much more quickly than they did prior to the injury. The good news is that these impairments can improve with direct and indirect interventions.

CHAPTER 14

MARITAL AND FAMILY CONCERNS

"God bless my wife. When I was crazy with grief and having an emotional breakdown, she was my rock. It doesn't mean we didn't talk about divorce. It means that we chose each other despite all the misery."

—**Pete McGuyer**, U.S. Marine Chief Petty Officer, Reconnaissance and Marine Special Operations Command

"The longer you're in the operator family, the closer Operator Syndrome creeps into your own home. As spouses, we talk to one another about intimate struggles, because no one else quite understands the unique challenges we face. I've seen marriages destroyed, families torn apart, and guys completely lose themselves because of the negative impacts of Operator Syndrome: sleep disturbance that turn into self-medicating with alcohol, changes in guys' personalities and emotions that result in intense anger outbursts and abuse, and of course, suicide. It's not a matter of if you know someone affected, it's when."

—**Dr. Jennifer Byrne**, U.S. Air Force veteran, Special Operations spouse

"No matter how much you think you are shielding your children, you are not. They are having the same thoughts, and your feelings are contagious to them. Talk to your children!"

—**Leslie Luna**, U.S. Navy veteran, SEAL spouse

"I had a vision of one day ending my wars. I dreamt of coming home to a normal life with my wife and kids. But when the day arrived, I suddenly took notice of all the damage and destruction that had piled up around me. My wife and kids had built life-styles and norms without me, and they were used to having holidays and major life events without me present. Before my wife left me, she told me she had envisioned my funeral a hundred times. She was more tired than I was."

—**Mark Ozdarski**, U.S. Navy SEAL (Ret.)

"I promise you that your wife has a different concept of what your retirement will look like than you do. Your military time has been fulfilling for you, to a degree you have not yet comprehended. I describe it for most of us as similar to a Belgian Malinois dog, running hard and always looking for the next task to accomplish. Nothing makes you happier than that. But now that's it's over and you're done as a Barrel-Chested Freedom Fighter, your wife hopes you will sit on the couch and be a Basset Hound. She thinks you will simply turn off this thing that is your life. And I'm saying that that's not possible. If you plan to stay married, the two of you should talk about both your expectations."

—**Jason Beighley**, U.S. Army Sergeant Major (Ret.), Tier One Operator

"Operators' willingness to sacrifice for the sake of the people to their left and right overshadows their awareness of fundamental human needs like routine, celebration, tradition, play, and others. So, we break things down to one 'aha moment' at a time. Regular habits as simple as eating family dinner together, celebrating holidays and milestones, are incredibly powerful."

—**KaLea Lehman**, executive director and founder of the Military Special Operations Family Collaborative, U.S. Army Special Forces spouse

The lifestyle and profession of an operator is not exactly easy on a marriage or family. The frequent deployments, training evolutions, hazardous duties, long hours, chronic stress, injuries, uncertainty, constant potential for sudden death, and unit cultures are hard on intimate relationships and parenting. Divorce rates within the community are quite high, with very few marriages lasting. Many operators have had multiple marriages and divorces by the time they reach middle age.

Not only is the active-duty period of military service difficult, but the transition to civilian life post-service is also a serious challenge for many couples. Suddenly, the operator is home on a full-time, or at least more regular, basis. Household roles and expectations are likely to change, and adaptions are necessary for the entire family, at that point. In a 2023 podcast interview I conducted with Admiral Hendrickson for the Global SOF Foundation, he described this as an "accrued relationship debt."

On top of all of that, being an operator's spouse can be incredibly stressful, burdensome, lonely, and traumatic. It's certainly not easy functioning as a single parent.

Operator's spouses find themselves doing many of the following things:

- Planning their husband's funeral before a deployment
- Attending funerals for other operators or service members killed in action
- Wondering in a private moment if their husband is even alive
- Watching their children struggle, because their father is rarely home for birthdays, milestones, or holidays
- Crying privately because the man they married no longer even seems like the same person he was

There is another issue that doesn't get enough attention. Being married to an operator is isolating and lonely. Who can a spouse confide in apart from other spouses in the community? Typically, they find that people from outside of the SOF community have little understanding of their lives and experiences. That dividing line is made even wider by the sensitive nature of the operator's military work.

Yet another major issue for spouses and families is Operator Syndrome itself. The complex and severe injuries sustained by most operators compound all of the other challenges to marriage and parenting—and then some. Imagine living with a partner who doesn't sleep well, is constantly irritable and quick to anger, has difficulty with concentration and memory, is depressed, drinks too much, and seems to be struggling with secrets they won't or can't talk about. Many spouses say that having their operator at home is like having another child—a complicated child—to supervise and take care of.

Making efforts to communicate better, to collaborate in addressing Operator Syndrome, and to attend couples therapy, if necessary, can help lead to massive improvements in the relationship for the long term. I encourage couples to have hard and honest conversations with each other.

Men, in general, are in much better health when they include their spouses as full partners in their healthcare. This is a massively important aspect of overall health and wellness for the operator, and usually leads to a happier marriage and improved family relations all around.

Over the years, I've talked with several children of operators, and, of course, I've also heard about their experiences as seen through their parents' eyes. They tend to have a familiarity with death that separates them from most of their peers. Many grow up knowing about war, aware that a casualty affairs officer could show up at their home any time. They have attended funerals—five, ten, or even more—for men they knew as "uncles."

Some children describe this as a weight or a dark cloud that hangs over their lives. Some even report feeling guilty that while their father is deployed overseas, they are at home enjoying the comforts of modern life and childhood. More than one adolescent has expressed guilt and frustration at not being allowed to train and join their father on war zone deployments. Add to this the reality that the father is rarely home and routinely misses birthdays, holidays, concerts, sporting events, and other milestones.

The life of an operator's child can be confusing, lonely, and heavy.

Survey research conducted by KaLea Lehman and the Military Special Operations Family Collaborative (MSOFC) identified eight key "home front" challenges to the healthy functioning of operators and their families. These were found to be especially problematic when they become part of family life for two or more years. These unhealthy and unsustainable factors are:

1. Prolonged, unpredictable family routines
2. Ceasing family celebrations
3. No or few practiced family traditions
4. Skipping family vacations or working while on leave
5. Regularly skipping or avoiding family dinner
6. Avoidance of important conversations
7. Limited awareness of invisible wounds
8. Pessimism regarding military service and tradition

These are difficult challenges, but each one of them represents an opportunity, a target for change. Map them out and do the opposite. Develop family routines and traditions, celebrate milestones and accomplishments, prioritize family time at home and on vacation, stop avoiding hard conversations, and start having regular family dinners!

Further Recommended Readings
- *Arsenal of Hope: Tactics for Taking on PTSD, Together* by Jen Satterly and Holly Lorincz (Post Hill Press, 2021)
- *The Warrior's Table: Recipes that Cultivate Connection through War, Change, and Uncertainty* by The Cast Iron Crew, a.k.a. Military Special Operations Family Collaborative (Ballast Books, 2023)

CHAPTER 15

INTIMACY CONCERNS

"Sometimes I struggle with erectile dysfunction (ED)."
— **Anonymous** (said quietly by almost every operator ever)

"In order to allow his mind to submit to intimacy, he requires a disconnect from work and life distractions. That, paired with his physical exhaustion from years of endocrine and orthopedic exertion, takes a high degree of effort to find the space to connect. The desire is there, but I believe the expectation to perform is overwhelmed by a past filled by operating at the highest level. The intensity and self-induced pressure to complete as many daily tasks as possible play the most significant factors in his inability to shut down his mind and reignite his emotional and physical intimacy."
— **Jana Rutherford**, spouse of former U.S. Navy SEAL

"When I think about cancer in Special Operations Forces—alongside the challenges of TBI, PTSD, suicide, and other chronic medical issues common to the community, and even transition

out of the military—I see a thread running through all of them: isolation. In response to our need to be seen as—at our best—in control, strong, healthy, and able, we self-isolate and enter our own rat hole where we address or live with our issues 'by self.' It's ironic how the best teammates in the world don't depend upon the team when they need it the most. We armor up and shield ourselves even from those who would lay down their lives for us. We all need to find a new level of vulnerability and openness that allows us to expose our humanity, (in our own mind) expose 'our weaker selves.' We need to be present with teammates and loved ones in a space that focuses on the mission of healing—and let go of managing perception and ego. Most of us lack the training and experience to do that well, but even doing it poorly is better—better for body, mind, heart, and soul—than fighting alone."

—**Rob Newson**, U.S. Navy SEAL (Ret.)

They had been married for just over eighteen years and their two children were well into their teenage years. He was a retired operator, starting his own business, and she was a freelance graphic designer. Their life together so far had been remarkably happy and free of conflict or drama. There was no infidelity, or even accusations of infidelity.

And yet something was wrong.

She said he was "checked out," "distant," no longer sweet and considerate like he had been during their courtship and the first fifteen years of their marriage. Most of the time he was silent and brooding.

He said he was exhausted all the time and frustrated that the house and children required so much of his time and effort. Because she often brought up the idea of moving to a more expensive neighborhood, he thought she lacked appreciation for all that he had provided.

Both agreed they had not made much room for intimacy in their marriage. Since the first child had been born, there had been no vacations or even weekend getaways for just the two of them. It had been years since there had even been a date night.

Did they cuddle on the couch while watching movies? No.

Did they ever take a walk and hold hands? No.

How often did they make love? Neither could remember the last time.

What did they talk about? Work, house chores, challenges with the children.

He was exasperated that she didn't do more of the housework and shuttling of the children to and from school. Sometimes she didn't even get out of bed until eight or nine o'clock in the morning.

She knew that a lot of the other operators had affairs or left their wives for other women. There was no evidence that her husband was unfaithful, but she couldn't help but wonder. She had snooped through his phone several times, but found nothing suspicious.

He acknowledged that he was lonely, that he missed the people he served with and didn't feel he could talk openly to his wife. When he had tried previously, she had shut him down, telling him there wasn't much point to talking about the distant past.

She wanted him to be the way he "used to be."

He wondered if maybe she was depressed, but she refused to consider the possibility.

Even when they were seated on the couch beside each other in their living room, there was a distance between them.

They didn't make eye contact with or touch each other. There was no tenderness in the air.

She asked the question they were each privately grappling with: "How can we recover the contentment and the intimacy we used to share?"

———————

Combat soldiers—warriors—have long been famous for their stoicism. They have seen and done things most of us have not. They can be hard to read, hard for civilians to relate to. Even their spouses and families are likely to describe them as aloof, distant, and certainly not the same as they used to be. But intimacy matters to humans. We need it, crave it, and our success in long-term relationships depends upon it. It is very common for operators to have difficulty with both emotional and sexual intimacy.

Emotional Intimacy

We are social creatures by nature, evolved from small hunter-gatherer tribes, interdependent for survival. This means humans, as a species, are designed to thrive on positive connections with other humans they trust, and they suffer profoundly when they do not have these connections.

Operators experience an intense and unique emotional intimacy with their brothers-in-arms. They train, travel, live, and fight together, usually in close quarters. Violence, death, and killing—as harrowing as they are—can also bring profoundly intimate moments.

Nothing can replace the military brotherhood after an operator steps away from it. This is one reason that leaving military service can be an extraordinarily lonely and painful transition period. Substance abuse, excessive pornography, or infidelity can each represent massive barriers to both emotional and sexual intimacy. Be mindful of this as you make that transition.

It is critical that operators allow themselves to seek, open up to, and allow for intimacy and affection. This is unfamiliar territory for many guys, and they probably haven't had the chance to learn and develop the emotional social skills that it takes. As an operator restored to his civilian relationships, you need to try anyway. Social skills, like any other skills, can be learned with regular effort, practice, and feedback.

Make an effort to meet other people and be open to making friends. Search for those meaningful emotional connections, not just superficial ones. Friendships don't have to be purely instrumental connections that facilitate work or business. Seek out people who might be different from you.

Identify the important relationships already in your life and have honest, deep conversations on a regular basis, even if you have to schedule them. A twenty-second quiet hug with someone you love can be magical because it releases oxytocin chemicals into the bloodstream.

You couldn't survive alone in the military. Don't try to go it alone now that you are home. A famous poem by John Donne (1571–1631)—himself a combat soldier, priest, and scholar—says it far, far better than I ever possibly could:

> No man is an island,
> Entire of itself,
> Every man is a piece of the continent,
> A part of the main.

If a clod be washed away by the sea,
Europe is the less.
As well as if a promontory were.
As well as if a manor of thy friend's
Or of thine own were:
Any man's death diminishes me,
Because I am involved in mankind,
And therefore never send to know for whom the bell tolls;
It tolls for thee.

Sexual Intimacy

Research shows that veterans, as a group, are at an increased risk for sexual dysfunction relative to the general population, especially if they have PTSD. It is very common for operators to have difficulty with physical affection and sexual intimacy. There are many reasons for this, but before we get into them, let's acknowledge that we live in a society where frank conversations about sexual health are not easy. Troubles in this area are often not discussed.

We know that TBI can affect endocrine levels, such as testosterone. It is very common for operators to experience low testosterone, which has obvious consequences for sexual functioning. Furthermore, many other difficulties operators face can contribute to sexual dysfunction or problems with intimacy.

These include the following:

- Pain
- Insomnia or sleep deprivation
- Anger and rage
- Depression
- Anxiety

- Alcohol abuse
- PTSD
- Trust issues
- Medication side effects and multidrug interactions
- Effects of natural aging

In addition to this list, there is also potentially a dark side that contributes to sexual dysfunction. Research indicates that military populations in general have higher rates of domestic violence, risky sexual behaviors, and sexually transmitted diseases. We all know that operators are not "choir boys," and we wouldn't want them to be. Most will already know that within the culture of some units, there is a certain acceptance of pornography and infidelity—both of which can be addictive and usually lead to immense levels of shame and guilt.

In addition to *all* of that, we have to be mindful of relationship dynamics and the fact that being the partner or spouse of an operator brings its own challenges. Emotional intimacy between an operator and his partner can be strained and challenged by their previous career lifestyles and accumulated experiences of service life, as well as by the potential conflict emerging from that, often leading to years of marital dissatisfaction.

So, how can you improve your sexual functioning? Obviously, the answer will vary by individual, and I can only offer some general thoughts and suggestions.

Treatment for TBI, low testosterone, insomnia, pain, depression, and everything else covered in this book should lead to benefits in romantic relationships, sexual health, and emotional intimacy. Lifestyle and behavioral habits should also play a powerful role. Anything that is good for the heart is good for sexual performance; that means regular exercise, a healthy diet, quality sleep, relaxation and recovery, and moderation in substance use.

Intimacy problems are tough ones, and modern medicine really doesn't have many answers, but simply making a conscious, concerted effort to change can pay off big time—and it usually does.

CHAPTER 16

MILITARY-TO-CIVILIAN TRANSITION CONCERNS

"I remember the day I left the Marine Special Operations Command (MARSOC) compound. It felt like a messy breakup. I cried because I didn't know any other way to express how I felt."
—**Pete McGuyer**, U.S. Marine Chief Petty Officer, Reconnaissance and MARSOC

"Leaving active service was like divorcing all my friends simultaneously. They kept living their close-knit lives, and I only had memories to hold onto. Even those who continued to be part of my life were building new stories without me; that was hard."
—**Lisa Jaster**, U.S. Army Reserve Lieutenant Colonel, partner and senior contributor at Talent War Group, author of *Delete the Adjective: A Soldier's Adventures in Ranger School*

"Leaving the community I had been a part of my entire adult life was intimidating. I felt like the world outside of the military had very little genuine purpose. I had to learn to appreciate I still had a lot to offer people, and a lot of the same things that bound

my teammates and I together existed outside; it just looked a little different. The focus shifted from my team to my family."
   —**Chad White**, U.S. Army Special Forces Sergeant
First Class (Ret.)

"Watching your spouse transition is like watching someone grieve the death of their spouse. But instead, it's the death of their own life. The one they once knew. Watching them move through the stages of grief opens many progression opportunities, but only when they're ready. I find offering supportive care for a transitioned operator is often like conversing with a foreigner. He's starting to understand his new land, but often romances the fond memories of the way he used to live."
   —**Corrie Burton**, U.S. Army Special Forces fiancée

*"My experience and my observation of other vets I know are that perhaps the biggest challenge post-military is to recalibrate your personal identity. You did not '**do the job**' of an assaulter or combat medic, you actually '**were**' an assaulter or combat medic. This difference in how we perceive ourselves is key to understanding our path forward, and to help us normalize our life after we no longer are what we did."*
   —**Jason Beighley**, U.S. Army Sergeant Major (Ret.),
Tier One Operator

"I never imagined that getting out was going to be more difficult than being in and deploying into combat and dealing with the stress of never knowing what your life is going to be like year to year. Transitioning was the hardest part about the military for me. I lost my mind in the process about two years out of the military and on about twelve-plus meds from the VA, I lost it. I didn't want to be here anymore. I luckily found a network of healers and got introduced to DMT therapy. 5-MeO-DMT saved my life and changed

my life. I have not drunk alcohol or taken pills since September 9, 2019, when I did my first psychedelic assisted therapy."

—**Prime Hall**, former U.S. Marine Raider

"The transition we experienced exiting the military was highly chaotic. Being in special operations for years had provided many amazing opportunities for my husband, but transitioning into the civilian world was not something he had prepared for and when it was thrust upon him it required him to dig deep into what this new future was going to look like."

—**Andrea Gallagher**, U.S. Navy SEAL spouse,
president of The Pipe Hitter Foundation

"If we approach our transition out of the military in the same way we prepared for selection, we'll be successful. When we half-ass it, we end up on our asses. Transition is a lifelong deployment with a new indig."

—**Herb Thompson**, U.S. Army Special Forces 5th
Group Team Sergeant (Ret.), author of *The Transition
Mission*

I magine if someone like me, a civilian, a professional, was forced into a "transition" away from the life I have lived for my entire adult life. In this hypothetical scenario, I am no longer a psychologist, and my PhD becomes meaningless.

I'm now required to relocate to a new land, a new culture. I find myself in a country where, yes, they might speak English and pop culture, the internet, and other media are all pretty much the same as they always have been. But the language as spoken by the people I meet, even though it is in English, is difficult to understand. Words mean the same thing, but often they mean other things too. Customs are very different. Most of the people around me have no understanding of what I spent the past several decades doing. I am as much a stranger to them as they are to me.

In essence, I am required to start over again. I have to learn new skills and find a new way to earn a living. Maybe I have a small amount of savings or monthly pension income, but it's not enough and even if it were, I'm too young to sit around a house with nothing purposeful to do with myself. There is both a financial pressure and a strong need to do work that feels meaningful to me. How do I find that combination? Most of the new types of jobs I hear about (or even try) seem boring and empty.

I miss my "tribe." The people I worked with all those years are still available by phone if I feel up to calling them, but I no longer interact with them in the course of my daily activities. They are far away, both literally and figuratively. Many are still on the other side of the transition, still functioning as professionals with no thought to me or what I might be doing now. To them, I have disappeared. The others—the ones who have already transitioned themselves—are spread to the wind. I am lonely and doubting myself.

There are new unspoken rules and etiquette that I have to somehow pick up on and incorporate into my new identity. I am naïve and nobody in my new world even thinks to explain these new rules to me, in part because they have no reference point to where I came from. It's not their fault, but they frustrate me, nevertheless. Often, I pull away from them and isolate myself so that I can better relax and clear my head.

Gradually I start to realize that a handshake in my new world doesn't mean the same thing as it did in my prior world. Trusting others is now a lot harder, because I don't know who they are or where they come from. We have few shared experiences. We may live in the same neighborhood or work in the same place, but that doesn't mean their larger goals are the same as mine. It seems really complicated.

I have to develop a short narrative to explain my past life to people in my new one. I don't know how to dress myself anymore, because different clothing is supposed to be worn on different occasions, and I have trouble discerning the standards of the new society I live within. Maybe I make an effort to blend in, but mostly it's easier to do my thing and not mingle too much with this new society.

Personal values seem to be different. Hard work, sacrifice, cooperation, and loyalty all seem to be defined in ways I don't understand. The people around me, while not necessarily malicious, don't seem serious or dedicated enough, at least not in the way I expect of others. In fact, many people are frivolous, wasteful, and lazy. They don't appreciate how good they have it. I don't understand them, and their behaviors often anger me. So, I withdraw further.

Apply all that to yourself. Now add on the reality that you have injuries other people cannot see and do not understand. It's much harder to learn new material and master new skills than it used to be. This is frustrating, because you used to be excellent at everything you set out to do. You were an elite performer in a very challenging career environment. Now you sometimes feel like an ignorant klutz. Sometimes people stare at you funny, especially if they learn where you come from. They have stereotypes about you that are generally rather negative and usually very wrong. While they may express respect, their nonverbal signals often scream fear.

Lastly, you no longer have a governing authority to guide you. You have to seek out and find that element for yourself.

Where do you go? When do you go there? What do you do when I arrive? There are new freedoms and opportunities, but even these are confusing. Suddenly you have so many more choices to make. This is extremely stressful, and nobody else understands that. There are very few people that you can trust to guide you.

Where do you even start with this transition that has been forced upon you?

This is how I explain the military-to-civilian transition.

It's beyond the scope of this chapter, of this book even, to provide real guidance on how to best manage your transition. In a perfect world, soldiers would start preparing two years prior to leaving the service. Obviously, this is often not possible. But understand that the transition is a major challenge for virtually every operator who goes through it. It will be far more difficult, more stressful than you expect. There are books, programs, coaches, and foundations that can help. Seek them out and be patient with yourself and your family. Accept that the process may take two to five years post-service. Also accept that you may never fully be a "regular citizen" again – and that's okay.

Further Recommended Readings

- *The Transition Mission: A Green Beret's Approach to Transition from Military Service* by Herb Thompson (SF2BIZ, 2019)
- *Wounding Warriors: How Bad Policy is Making Veterans Sicker and Poorer* by Daniel Gade and Daniel Huang (Ballast Books, 2021)

CHAPTER 17

TOXIC EXPOSURE ILLNESSES AND CANCERS

"War is toxic and its history reveals a troubling pattern. From Vietnam to Desert Storm to the War on Terrorism, we see a pattern of disbelief, denial, and delay. This is justified by an insistence on research and irrefutable evidence that often lags by decades. We've also seen how comprehensive and responsive medical policy and programs save lives and their delay in approval and implementation squanders lives. It's well past time for leaders and policy makers to move from skepticism to belief and active assistance. We are blessed with enormous opportunity: social media and numerous communication channels to inform and educate those at risk; genetics and AI to fast-track research; immunotherapy to individualize cancer care and cure; precision nutrition and metabolic treatment; and a wealth of nonprofit and commercial organizations that can partner and innovate until the government swings into action. The tool kit is ready. We cannot wait."

—**Rob Newson**, U.S. Navy SEAL (Ret.)

I don't have the medical or scientific background to even begin to do this chapter justice, and even if I did, I would have to write an entire book. But one problem we face is that we don't have very good data on the prevalence of toxic exposure illness or cancers, for either GWOT veterans generally or the SOF community specifically. SOCOM has held at least one recent forum in 2021 on cancer in the SOF community to discuss the possibility of conducting epidemiological or medical surveillance research. Many of those who attended viewed this conference as a potential start to considering the problem, but only just that. It's not clear that any progress has been made since.

Here's a stark anecdote I previously alluded to in Chapter 1 that demonstrates this exposure: Two operators I know independently reported spending time at a secret military site formerly established and used by the Soviet Union. They described "green pools" on the ground all around and even inside the perimeter of this camp. Neither one had any idea what the green muck was, but it was almost certainly not benign. Operators have often had to spend time during their careers in these questionable environments potentially rife with toxicity.

———

Toxic exposures for soldiers are not limited to burn pits. They also include fuel, diesel exhaust, ammunition, explosives, heavy metals, radiofrequency, radiation, depleted uranium, asbestos, toluene, benzene, air pollution, small particulate matter, contaminated food and water sources, smoke, carbon monoxide, carbon dioxide, oxygen-deficient environments, microbiological viruses, electromagnetic energy, and others.

The extreme heat in Iraq, for example, could melt down flame-retardant chemicals in uniforms that might then be absorbed directly into the skin. This parallels recent findings that the bunker gear protective equipment used by firefighters is also often toxic.

Collectively these exposures can cause a wide range of health problems, including brain injury, neurological damage, pulmonary disorders, autoimmune disorders, and cancers. Our failure to understand toxic exposures in service members means that we are behind the curve on screening, early identification, proper diagnoses, and effective and timely treatments. Too often physical symptoms are dismissed as "psychosomatic" by medical providers, cueing up a referral for mental health treatment. By the time a veteran's cancer is finally recognized, it can be too late.

The VA's list of "presumptive" cancers qualified for service connection include those found in the following parts of the body: brain, head, ears, eyes, mouth, neck, throat, nasal area, spinal cord, gastrointestinal region, and kidneys. In addition, the accepted list includes lymphoma, melanoma, reproductive cancer, and respiratory cancer. But many cancers are not on the "presumptive" list, including leukemia, bone cancer, and myeloproliferative neoplasms (which are a type of blood cancer).

What can you do?

Stay on top of regular physical exams. Get tested for heavy metals. Watch for signs and symptoms of potential illness, such as chronic fatigue, shortness of breath while exercising, severe unexplainable pain, loss of hair, and any other unusual indications.

If you have blood in your stool, chronic diarrhea, other gastrointestinal (GI) distress, unexplained weight loss, or are over forty-five, request a colonoscopy (and get tested for parasites and H. pylori bacteria, which are potential noncancerous causes of chronic GI distress). Colon cancer is treatable, but outcomes are far better if identified at an early stage.

Time is of the essence for most cancers. For this reason, consider undergoing cancer screening tests like the Galleri, which looks for fifty different types of cancer.

Finally, contact a VA Environmental Health Coordinator to learn more information about your potential exposures, schedule an exam, and possibly join one or more of the VA's six environmental health registries.

Stay alert and be proactive with your health.

CHAPTER 18

EXISTENTIAL CONCERNS

"As an operator, I knew my purpose, team, and identity. After retiring, I realized I had to find a new purpose and team while discovering my identity. Nothing would match the exhilaration and criticality of what I did on missions. If I sought out something similar, I'd fail. Changing my mindset that things would be different and that's ok was critical."

—**Herb Thompson**, U.S. Army Special Forces 5th Group Team Sergeant (Ret.), author of *The Transition Mission*

"Operators sacrifice so much of their body, mind, and soul to be on an assault team; the investment becomes supreme to all other things. They feel privileged to be a part of such an important tribe and mission. The mission always comes first above all else, including family and self. But after so much sacrifice, injury, and seeing so much gore and inhumanity, one must have a higher power to keep things in balance and continue. There must be a purpose."

—**Mark Ozdarski**, U.S. Navy SEAL (Ret.)

"Trying to fit all warriors into the typical DSM PTSD paradigm or blaming violence is totally out of touch with who we are. The absence of mission, the loss of brothers and sisters, the frustrations of civilian society are what strain the mind for many of us. Without intending to sound callous, the violence is not what bothers me; it is not the reason many are angry or short with people. When one spends years in a never-ending life or death situation, perspective changes. There's a lifting of the veil of life, and perhaps this heightened sense is stuck in drive. I and many others would do it again!"

—**Aric Gray**, U.S. Army Special Forces (Ret.), director of the Office of Protective Medicine, U.S. Department of State

"When working with operators, it is tempting to draw a straight line between combat trauma and Operator's Syndrome. However, adverse childhood events and trauma often echo through current symptoms and stress. By my count, 70 to 80 percent of those I treated had something chasing them from the past."

—**J. Christopher Fowler**, PhD, professor of psychology in psychiatry and behavioral health at Houston Methodist Hospital Behavioral Health

In the year 410 A.D., a Visigoth army led by King Alaric laid siege to Rome, finally entering the city when the Salarian Gate was left open in what was probably an act of betrayal. For three days the Germanic tribesman pillaged the city, raping, torturing, robbing, and murdering the people within its walls. Civilians, children, slaves, and aristocrats were all savaged. When the Visigoths left, they took with them all of the silver, gold, and precious jewels they could find. They also took human captives, some of whom would be ransomed, while others would be kept or sold into slavery.

In 1937, after taking the Chinese city of Nanking, the conquering Imperial Japanese Army committed mass rape, murder, torture, arson, and looting as part of a massacre of civilians and soldiers that lasted for six weeks. Estimates of the "Rape of Nanking" suggest the Japanese Army murdered at least two hundred thousand and raped twenty thousand.

Conquering armies throughout human history have often behaved thus.

People are killed in war, sometimes in astonishing numbers. The Mongol invasion of the Punjab ended in 1298 when twenty thousand Mongols were killed in one day of battle. The wounded were beheaded where they lay, while other survivors were taken to Delhi where they were publicly trampled to death by elephants.

At the Battle of Agincourt in 1415, over six thousand French troops were killed on the field, many of them under a shower of arrows. The Battle of Gettysburg in 1863 resulted in forty-five thousand casualties for both sides combined, although some estimates surpass fifty thousand. In 1864, the Union Army suffered seven thousand casualties at Cold Harbor within the first thirty minutes of their frontal assault on Confederate lines. On the first day of the Normandy Invasion on July 6, 1944, the Allies sustained 4,414 killed in action; later that year, they suffered nineteen thousand losses during the Battle of the Bulge, between December 1944 and January 1945.

The atomic bombs dropped on Hiroshima and Nagasaki in 1945 resulted in 130,000 to 220,000 deaths, mostly civilians. The months-long Siege of Baghdad in 1258 resulted in an estimated two million casualties—again, most of whom were civilians. The Battle of Stalingrad had an estimated 2.5 million casualties.

War is monstrous.

The Holocaust. The "Killing Fields" of Cambodia from 1975 to 1979. The 1994 Rwandan genocide, with eight hundred thousand killed in one hundred days. The Armenian genocide from 1915 to 1917. The Holdomor—Stalin's intentionally created famine that killed an estimated 3.5 to five million Ukrainian citizens between 1932 and 1933. Mao's "Great Leap Forward" from 1958 to 1962 led to an estimated fifty-five million deaths, primarily through starvation.

During the thirteenth century, the Mongol invasions of Eurasia resulted in the violent deaths of forty to one hundred million people. This was probably more than 10 percent of the entire human population on earth at the time. The An Lushan Rebellion from 755 to 763—a civil war attempting to overthrow the Tang Dynasty—resulted in an estimated thirty-six million deaths, up to two thirds of the total Chinese population.

The European powers' conquests of territory in South America, North America, and Africa resulted in tens of millions killed through war, famine, and disease. The Spanish Conquistadors wrested control of most of South America in the early sixteenth century, causing an estimated twenty million deaths, mostly due to yellow fever. Up to 95 percent of the indigenous population was wiped out as a consequence.

Military forces have committed atrocities, crimes against humanity, often on a colossal scale. Estimates suggest about half a million "gladiators" perished in the Colosseum across six centuries of Roman world dominance. After crushing the Spartacus-led slave rebellion between 73 and 71 BC, the Roman general Marcus Crassus ordered six thousand surviving slaves to be crucified to death along both sides of the Appian Way, from Naples to Rome—140 miles. Their tortured bodies were left to rot in the sun for all to see.

Military societies throughout history have practiced human sacrifice and cannibalism, from Egypt under the pharaohs to Hawaii before the arrival of Captain Cook and other European explorers and missionaries in the late eighteenth century. The Aztecs are thought to have sacrificed over one million people on their altars, including an estimated eighty thousand in 1487.

Horrific practices continue. Even today, many countries and militant groups around the world use fighters so young that Western democracies consider them to be children. "Child soldiers" are typically kidnapped, brainwashed, and forced to participate in executing and torturing prisoners, sometimes even their own parents, as part of their initiation.

America has its own history of brutality and war crimes. The GWOT included the mistreatment of prisoners in Abu Ghraib and the massacre of civilians in Haditha. If we look back further in our history, we see institutionalized slavery, the Andersonville Prison, Sherman's march to the sea, Wounded Knee, Fort Pillow, Balangiga in the Philippines, the fire-bombing of Dresden, No Gun Ri in Korea, My Lai in Vietnam, and many other incidents.

During the years I worked at the VA, from 1991 to 2006, my patients were mostly veterans of World War II, Korea, Vietnam, and Desert Storm. Many of them described witnessing and committing atrocities that would shock middle America. Some recounted such events without emotion, others through heaving sobs. Almost to a man, they acknowledged they had never spoken of these experiences with anyone after coming home.

Since the GWOT our enemies in Iraq and Afghanistan have often resorted to ancient barbaric practices, including crucifixion, stonings, beheadings, mounting heads for public display, violently raping children, women, and men, using children as shields or suicide bombers, enslaving women and children, torturing family members, executing prisoners, and many other brutalities I don't need to list. I've heard accounts of these horrors by American service members who witnessed them—often in real-time via live video surveillance feeds.

Sometimes American soldiers responded in kind.

———

And yet. The three largest Abrahamic religions—Judaism, Christianity, and Islam—share the common perspective that human life involves a choice between good and evil as dictated by divine law. The Ten Commandments given to Moses (known as Prophet Musa in Islam) on Mount Sinai are a list of God's inviolable laws and are fundamental aspects of Judaism, Christianity, and Islam. You probably already know them:

1. Thou shalt have no other gods before me.
2. Thou shalt not make unto thee any graven image.
3. Thou shalt not take the name of the Lord thy God in vain.
4. Remember the sabbath day, to keep it holy.
5. Honor thy father and thy mother.
6. Thou shalt not kill.
7. Thou shalt not commit adultery.
8. Thou shalt not steal.

9. Thou shalt not bear false witness against thy neighbor.
10. Thou shalt not covet.

Common to virtually every ancient civilization and major world religion—Judaism, Christianity, Islam, Buddhism, Hinduism, Taoism, Zoroastrianism—is some variation of what we refer to as the Golden Rule: *Do unto others as you would have them do unto you.* This concept of reciprocity requires a level of empathy, the ability to compassionately understand and honor the perspectives and rights of others.

Most religions allow for the concept of "righteous" killing, often including combat, self-defense (especially of one's home and family), and capital punishment for violent crimes. The "just war" doctrine is thought to be as old as warfare itself, though Augustine of Hippo first used the phrase and wrote about it in *The City of God* from 426 AD. For Augustine, an early Christian theologian, Christians should be pacifists—although war could be necessary and just if it was defensive in nature and fought to restore long-term peace. Writing over a thousand years later, Thomas Aquinas, in his *Summa Theologicae* from 1485, expanded on Augustine's writings in an effort to outline a framework and the necessary principles of a "just" war.

In the twentieth century, the Geneva Conventions of 1929 and 1949 were drafted to define basic rights of prisoners, civilians, and soldiers in war. They established an ethical and legal framework of protections afforded to noncombatants in a war zone, as well as protections for wounded or captured combatants. They have been formally ratified by 196 countries, covering almost the entire world. The Geneva Protocol from 1925 prohibits the use of biological and chemical weapons in war.

The historical record of war throughout human history shows that the "just" war conventions are not followed by all belligerents. This means that honorable soldiers in war will inevitably be confronted with situations, choices, and actions that profoundly conflict with the collective religious, moral, and legal values of human society.

———

Combat inevitably means killing, which is almost certainly the greatest taboo of all human behaviors. Soldiers also face a wide range of related existential issues that can have lasting effects on them.

The "fog of war," especially that of modern war with its long-range killing, has led to incidents of "friendly fire," or "blue on blue." During the airborne invasion of Sicily in July 1943, Allied naval gunners and shore batteries misidentified and fired on Allied C-47s crossing overhead from North Africa. Of 144 transport planes, twenty-three were shot out of the sky and thirty-seven more sustained heavy damage. American casualties, most from the 82nd Airborne Division, included eighty-eight killed in action, sixty-nine missing in action, and 162 wounded in action. Apart from its scale, this is not an isolated incident.

Soldiers throughout our species' history of warfare have always been confronted with the specter of their own death, the violent death of comrades, the aftermath of atrocities, impossible choices in combat such as attacking positions that may hold civilians, failures to act or errors that lead to the deaths of others, changing places or roles with another soldier who later dies in the subsequent operation, and being betrayed by their own nation and the society they fought for.

Even when it is fought righteously, war has always been—and continues to be—deeply horrifying.

Prototypical categories of existential concerns faced by operators and many other combatants during the GWOT include, but are almost certainly not limited to, the following:

- **The horror of killing other humans.** The taking of a human life is surely the most prohibited of all human behaviors. In his seminal book *On Killing*, Lieutenant Colonel David Grossman writes that the act of killing is so extremely traumatic for most soldiers that there is a deeply ingrained instinct not to do it, even when the soldier is in immediate danger of being killed himself. While the combat studies his conclusion is based on have been criticized, there is no doubt that modern military training uses exercises and customs intended to override this reluctance and desensitize trainees to killing the enemy. This is especially true in special operations.
- **The thrill of killing other humans.** In his 1936 short story "On the Blue Water," Ernest Hemingway wrote, "There is no hunting like the hunting of man, and those who have hunted armed men long enough and liked it, never care for anything else thereafter." In my most intimate conversations with operators, many have confidentially confided—usually something they've never told anyone outside their closest comrades—that they enjoyed it and now miss it. Many

don't regret killing enemies, saying instead they only wish they had killed more of them. More than one guy has told me about the ecstasy of killing a man with bare hands, or using a hammer, knife, hatchet, or whatever tool was handy. The feel, the smell, the heat, the sights and sounds, and the raw internal emotional arousal all contribute to the intensity of the experience. I also suspect a taste for killing is more common than we realize, a fact which naturally evokes an ongoing, soul-doubting dilemma. Even given the most "just" of operational careers, how do you reconcile killing men, enjoying it at the time, and missing it still today with the conflicting reality that you remain tethered to a Judeo-Christian-Islamic prohibition against killing?

- **Impossible choices.** All soldiers on or near the battlefield will face difficult, often impossible choices. Wartime situations and environments are volatile, uncertain, complex, and ambiguous. Decisions are often made under extreme pressure, with rushing adrenaline and only split seconds to decide. It is impossible to make the "right" call every single time. Should you pull the trigger? Fire on a target with potential for civilian casualties? Shoot an approaching woman or child? Protect a local if it risks the lives of comrades or operational security? Sacrifice your own life to save a comrade? Perform a "mercy" killing? There are no do-overs in combat.

- **Loss, grief, rage.** Casualties are unavoidable in war. Soldiers are grievously wounded, killed, or go missing. Intense training evolutions involving demolitions, parachuting, diving, helicopters, physical exhaustion, etc., are inherently dangerous and also lead to casualties. Because operators have exponentially more training and combat deployments and missions than most service members, over the course of decades, they have likely lost many, many comrades. This means a steady beat of ramp ceremonies, funerals, casualty affairs duties, and attending to Gold Star families. It also means a flow of grief and rage, for which there is little time to contemplate because of the high op tempo. That next mission, next training evolution, and next ridgeline don't leave much room for emotions in the moment. Operators are masters at compartmentalizing their feelings in order to maintain "front sight focus." However, they are often unprepared for the tidal wave of complex unresolved emotions when they finally do step away from the military.

- **Guilt, "moral injury," shame, "survivor's guilt."** Killing, accidents, failures to act, errors, surviving when others didn't, sins of omission, impossible choices, atrocities—soldiers must live with their past actions, and many remain tormented for years after their service. There is no easy formula for reconciling the deeply ingrained imperative not to kill with the realities of a horrific war. The death or torment of a young child in a war zone is probably the most common event that haunts soldiers. In the GWOT, U.S. soldiers saw children brutalized by insurgents, indigenous communities, and even their own parents. How many operators look at their own children now and see the eyes of a mortally wounded child who died in their arms? How do operators respond to their own children when asked questions about the war—when asked if they ever killed someone? Recently, one of my friends, a guy who is highly productive and still an elite performer in civilian life, wrote to me the following: "Here I am, a somewhat broken human being with lots of questions for the powers-that-be about why I went and slaughtered our 'enemies.' Why, oh why, was it okay to see the atrocities and even commit some myself in the name of self-preservation and mission first? How could I ever explain that to my son, or to society as a whole?"

- **Loss of empathy.** Involvement with war, especially over time, leads to a desensitization toward human suffering, injury, and death. Seeing the fiftieth violently killed human body does not affect a man as much as seeing the first one. With repetition—with exposure over time—the impact lessens. There is also a habituation to extreme danger to oneself. Operators can get used to the idea of their own death. If death becomes mundane, how does one maintain empathy beyond that point?

- **Loss of faith in God and in humanity.** Recently, a devoutly religious friend called me from deployment on the other side of the globe. In our conversation, he told me that his base was "not a target-rich environment for Christianity." Has there ever been a combat soldier who didn't wonder in despair, "*How could God allow this to happen?*" Many, if not all, combatants find their faith in God radically affected by war. How could they not? For some it means a strengthening of faith. For others it means questioning beliefs, or even a loss of faith altogether. The realities of war may be experienced as a violation of God's commandments. How can that not have a profound effect in some way? Emotions of grief, rage, guilt, and shame—especially related to war experiences—have a powerful influence on how we view the world and the other people in it. Combatants have seen the absolute worst of human behavior on a large scale. They have also seen the absolute best of human behavior. Some describe this as having "seen Heaven and Hell at the same time." Many also refer to their war experiences as a "battle between Good and Evil." This inevitably affects the way soldiers see and relate to other members of their species.

- **End of service experiences.** A high percentage of military careers end on a lousy note. Acute and chronic injuries can lead to a forced medical retirement. For officers, failure to achieve a critical promotion is often a stopping-out point. Selection of operators to serve in Tier One units is highly competitive, with many elite candidates failing to make the cut. It is even somewhat common for guys to run afoul of their commanders or be ostracized by unit mates, leading to an abrupt and unhappy departure from that command. In 2016, I attended the celebration event of a friend who was retiring from the Navy after almost thirty years of service. It was held at the SEAL Heritage Center at Little Creek Naval Base. While the ceremony was powerful and moving, I was surprised to be told that such observances were actually rather rare. Apparently—and this fits with what I have seen and heard since—very few operators choose to have any formally sponsored farewell. Some are too angry, and others just want to leave quietly to get on with their lives.

- **Loss of purpose and mission.** For operators after military service, there is often a feeling of numbness and emptiness toward the daily humdrum grind of civilian life and work, as well as a loss of empathy with the civilians themselves. Think back to the Hemingway quote from earlier in this list, about how hard it is to care for anything else after having "hunted armed men long enough and liked it." Operators volunteered for a career full of life-and-death moments. The work is physical, intellectual, and exhilarating. It involves sanctioned violence and powerful toys. You were surrounded by people you trusted, loved, and with whom you shared a mission. How easily can you sit behind a desk now for ten to twelve hours after that? Where do your elite skills of war fit in a peacetime job? Does the mission of your new employment, your new community, feel meaningful to you? Can you find others who will rise to the level of your standards? How do you handle the victim status conferred on you by a well-intentioned but ignorant society and VA system?

- **Loss of tribe.** Over tens of thousands of years, our ancestors evolved to be highly interdependent for survival. Everyone in the tribe had a role to play, and their existential challenges of survival bonded them together in a tight-knit group. They worked together, ate together, played together, slept together, and loved together. Nobody was ever alone. Calamity and good fortune alike were shared by all. Soldiers today experience this tribal life with their brothers-in-arms, their squad mates, and their units. For years, they work collaboratively with comrades who share their purpose, have similar training and mindsets, and consistently go the extra mile for the mission and for you. Very few humans today ever experience anything like this, so they don't know—they *can't* know—what it means. The military brotherhood is very difficult to replace after an operator leaves service. It's a special kind of loneliness. Most operators experience it as a sledge-hammer to the gut.

- **Childhood trauma.** Many of my colleagues and I have noted that a very high percentage of operators report extensive histories of childhood trauma. Many of those childhoods involved some combination of physical abuse, witnessed domestic violence, sexual abuse by parents and older siblings, parental neglect, early drug use, criminal activities and brushes with law enforcement, running with gangs, and poor scholastic performance. Many operators also acknowledge they were raised without a father figure. The military is one avenue toward effectively developing as a man, and special operations is a way to achieve excellence against all odds (and naysayers). Perhaps combat is a way to expunge old demons. Derek Nadalini, a retired U.S. Army Ranger and SMU operator, refers to this as the "ambition of shame." But what happens when the operator's career is over? Sometimes those childhood demons are still there, unresolved, and now the operator has time to contemplate and feel them. This can emerge as a toxic stew of unprocessed childhood and adult traumas, including loss, grief, rage, and anxiety.
- **National and societal betrayal.** After the war is over and the swords have been beaten back into

CHRIS FRUEH, PhD

ploughshares, soldiers and veterans are almost always left feeling betrayed by the nation and society they fought for. To varying degrees, this has been true in the aftermath of every significant American war, even going back as far as the nation's founding.

- **American Revolutionary War.** After the American Revolutionary War, officers were first granted a federal pension in 1781, while enlisted soldiers would not receive one until 1818—and only then if they were indigent. Service pensions for all enlisted soldiers were not granted until 1832—forty-nine years after the war ended.

- **World War I.** In 1932, twenty thousand unemployed veterans of World War I organized as the "Bonus Expeditionary Forces" and marched on Washington, DC, camping in shantytowns and demanding bonus payments they had been promised. After two months of stalemate, they were driven away by U.S. Army troops under the command of General Douglas MacArthur (along with Majors Dwight D. Eisenhower and George S. Patton). The troops advanced on unarmed veterans with fixed bayonets and tanks.

- **World War II.** During my years working at the VA Medical Center in Charleston, South Carolina from 1991 to 2006, I had the privilege to work with veterans from every era since the early 1940s. The World War II veterans, by then in their seventies or eighties, mostly scoffed at the idea that they had ever personally received a parade upon homecoming. Virtually all of them would tell you the American public has no idea about their actual wartime experiences and has little appreciation for how it affected them.

- **Vietnam War.** Aggrieved Vietnam War veterans commonly perceive that they won all their battles but lost the war because of weak national politicians and generals. Rules of engagement, logistics, and strategic decisions held them back. It was the first "TV war," with nightly footage of the day's most ghastly moments broadcast to the home front. The American public was horrified to see the actual realities of war in their living room every night. Many veterans and historians believe the sharp loss of public support is the reason the war was lost. This time, returning soldiers were spit upon and openly reviled by an angry segment of the U.S. population.

- **POWs.** Former prisoners of war have had additional frustrations. For several years around 2000, I had the privilege to work collaboratively with the South Carolina chapter of a national POW foundation on a small research project.[7] All but one of the former POWs were World War II veterans. I attended their monthly meetings, banquets, and an annual conference. They were resilient men, though also frustrated by a nation that didn't seem to remember their sacrifice. I also collaborated with Mike McGrath, then-president of NAM-POWs. Around that time, McGrath had written a letter to the secretary of the VA informing

---

7   Funded by the Center for Naval Analyses, Department of Defense (2001–2002)

him that the system seemed to have about ten thousand Vietnam-era POWs on its rolls nationally, when, in fact, there were only eight hundred POWs (662 military, 138 civilians) repatriated from Hanoi. McGrath could name every one of them from memory, in alphabetical order. He was angry that thousands of men were fraudulently receiving POW benefits from a VA that apparently didn't verify service records.

- **Global War on Terror.** The GWOT is no different. There are so many dispiriting elements of this prolonged conflict, I don't even know where to begin, but here are just a few issues that alienate and discourage service members: shifting rules of engagement; the first Iraq pullout that left the field open for ISIS to arise; after-action reports that covered up unpleasant truths; the military politics surrounding awards for valor; politicized military criminal justice prosecutions; exaggerated accusations of "white extremism" in the ranks; the DOD-wide vaccine mandate resisted by many service members; degraded military budgets; neglected technological capabilities; and the Kabul withdrawal and consequent abandonment of strategic territory, matériel, and—most importantly—allied Afghans, many of whom were closely connected to American operators. Books have and will continue to be written about these and other betrayals, but with the alleged "end" of the GWOT, U.S. politicians and citizens seem to have moved on. A nation indifferent to the sacrifice of its soldiers now appears to be following an agenda that seems deeply un-American to many operators, who see a country with a dropping workforce participation rate, declining religious faith, failing public schools, a divisive focus on identity politics, and an inability to meet the physical fitness requirements of military service. Throughout all of this, it is easy to wonder if a driving reason for war is power and money for an elite few. And from most operators, I often hear the following questions: "Is this what I fought for? Is this what my comrades died for?"

———

What does one do with existential burdens such as these? They don't lend themselves to medical interventions, or necessarily even to psychological ones. Combatants often have no one to talk to about these things. Understandably, they don't want to put terrible images into the minds of their civilian friends or family members. They also worry about legal repercussions. Few social workers and psychologists are well-prepared to listen or respond in useful ways. Some operators believe that only a higher power can help, and of these, some turn to religious or ecumenical counseling. Many operators have found peace through a psychedelic journey with ibogaine, 5-MeO-DMT, ayahuasca, or psylocibin. Still others claim benefit from ketamine infusion, an FDA-approved treatment for depression. Most also look outward, continuing their life of service to community.

———

This chapter was by far the hardest one for me to write. Although, as a civilian, I may lack confidence in my ability to address these issues usefully, or in a manner that is universally helpful, I will remind operators of this: you served for your comrades, your family, and your country, and your service carried the will and authority of a democratic nation behind it.

Please don't secretly hold on to the burden of existential angst alone. Plant a tree, say a prayer, or volunteer your time to a cause. Coach youth sports. Use your skills to help organizations that rescue victims of human trafficking. Try daily journaling. Adopt a dog or a cat. Join a softball league. Write a song. Resist the massive pull to numb yourself with alcohol or drugs. Don't compartmentalize and pretend the issues are not there. Try to find someone—friend, mentor, pastor, therapist—who you can open up to, even if just a little bit.

Further Recommended Readings
- *Man's Search for Meaning* by Victor Frankl (Beacon Press, 1959)
- *On Killing* by Lieutenant Colonel Dave Grossman (Back Bay Books, 1996)
- *Tribe: On Homecoming and Belonging* by Sebastian Junger (Twelve, 2016)

CHAPTER 19

SUICIDE

"I've had seven buddies eat a bullet after coming home."
—**Anonymous**, U.S. Marine Corps Force
Reconnaissance, private defense contractor

"What we didn't know was how twenty years of the GWOT op tempo would affect us long-term. Now we are seeing so many suicides and cancer deaths."
—**Geoff Dardia**, functional medicine certified health
coach, U.S. Army Special Forces Master Sergeant,
founder of the SOF Health Initiative Program

"I believe the suicide epidemic is due to falling away from your community and not having the true peer support to explain your thoughts and feelings without being judged."
—**Joey Fio**, former U.S. Navy SEAL, senior director
of health at the SEAL Future Foundation

"Operator Syndrome lays it all out to be understood. I spent twenty-five years in the Army with twenty-one being in special

operations. Frueh's work is spot on and describes the issues most of our Special Operations warrior families are facing. I spent most of my days considering taking my own life by suicide just to end the constant feelings of loss, embarrassment, shame, anger, rage, and constant conversations about how sorry I was for my actions. This led to the consistent realization that I was broken and needed to be removed from the society that I spent my life protecting. We are facing a nationwide epidemic of anger-related, rage-fueled outbursts from many of our Special Operations warriors who have no idea why they feel this way, and if they can't fix problems, they are trained to remove them. When you are the perceived problem, the idea of removal from society is first on the mind daily."

—**Tom Satterly**, U.S. Army Special Forces Command Sergeant Major (Ret.), CEO and cofounder of All Secure Foundation, author of *All Secure: A Special Operations Soldier's Fight to Survive on the Battlefield and the Homefront*

Military suicides, both during and after active service, have long been a concern of the U.S. Army—and, more recently, Veterans Affairs. Current evidence shows that twenty-two veterans die by suicide every day, while other research suggests the true number may be twice that. We don't really know. A precise estimate of suicides is difficult to come by, because there isn't a complete database or tracking of veterans in the U.S. The VA primarily compiles data on the veterans who use their system, and even for those, the tracking of deaths and causes of death can be complicated.

We often face the challenge of being able to know with certainty what a dead person's intent was. Is a death an accident or a suicide? This is especially true in single motor vehicle crashes and drug overdoses. A significant percentage of suspected suicides cannot be confirmed with a note, because there isn't one. We also rarely see any comparison of military suicides with civilian suicides. Therefore, we do not consider the full context when attempting to develop solutions to what we, at least rhetorically, identify as unacceptably high rates of military-related suicides.

My ongoing twelve-year collaboration with historian Jeff Smith and his academic colleagues has led to several recent insights based on historical records.[8] Suicide rates for active-duty U.S. Army soldiers have increased significantly since 2006 when compared to rates from 1900 to 1950, and they are surprisingly higher than those rates from even our country's deadliest war. During the Civil War, the Union Army documented a total of 278 suicides over the course of four years, resulting in an annual rate decidedly lower than the U.S. Army recorded during any year of the GWOT. Suicide rates do not seem to be driven primarily by combat experiences.

However, our examination of U.S. Army suicides dating back to 1817 revealed that these rates have fluctuated considerably over time, typically going *down* during active combat and *up* immediately *after* a major war. If this pattern holds, there may yet be a further rise in suicides in the coming years. Lastly, the suicide rate of soldiers historically parallels that of military-age male civilians. This suggests that causes of suicide are almost certainly multifactorial and driven by larger societal trends rather than by military stressors alone. U.S. Army and

---

8   Christopher Frueh and Jeffrey A. Smith, "Suicide, Alcoholism, and Psychiatric Illness among Union Forces during the U.S. Civil War," *Journal of Anxiety Disorders* 26 (2012): 769–775; Jeffrey A. Smith, et al, "A Historical Examination of Military Records of U.S. Army Suicide, 1819–2017," *JAMA Network Open* 2, no. 12 (2019): e1917448; Jeffrey A. Smith, et al, "A Historical Comparison of U.S. Army and U.S. Civilian Suicide Rates, 1900–2020," *Psychiatry Research* 323 (2023): 115182.

civilian males in the age groups of thirty-five to forty-four, forty-five to fifty-four, and fifty-five to sixty-four have increased substantially since 2006. This current spike may not be an aberration, but instead a sustained trend and return to "normal," at least historically speaking, after an unusually and consistently low rate for U.S. Army suicides from 1975 to 2004, during which rates for soldiers stabilized below civilian male rates.

Our team has not been able to obtain any administrative data on SOF suicides, active-duty or post-service. However, the special operations community is not immune to suicide. Nearly every operator I have talked to has acknowledged he has contemplated suicide (a.k.a. "suck-starting my pistol" or "levitating my Glock") at some point. Most of those suicidal moments involved a loaded pistol in hand with safety off. Every operator has comrades who have died by suicide. I hear about another operator suicide almost every month. Some of these incidents involve high-profile operators.

Mike Day died by suicide in 2023. He was a former Navy SEAL and Silver Star recipient who, in 2007, survived twenty-seven gunshot wounds while on target in Iraq and later wrote about resilience in his 2020 memoir. This suicide shook the community. When one of the toughest, most respected, badass guys takes his life, what hope is there for anyone else?

Most operators who killed themselves did so with a gunshot to the head. Others overdosed. Some have killed themselves in front of their wives and children, often in a moment of rage.

Thomas Joiner, a prominent psychological researcher who studies suicide, has a powerful theory. In his book *Why People Die by Suicide*, he theorizes that exposure to violence, death, and killing causes humans to become habituated (remember that word?) to death—the death of others as well as the idea of their own death.

How much death and killing have you seen? Have you visualized or meditated on your own death? How many times have you completed the pre-deployment plans for your own funeral? Once you accept the possible, or even probable, likelihood of your own death—as most operators learn to do—the notion of killing yourself may, tragically enough, seem an acceptable solution to intractable problems. According to Dr. Joiner's theory, this habituation to death is a major risk factor for suicide.

During a recent conversation I had with Chris Kurinec, a longtime U.S. Army Operational Detachment Alpha operator, he offered an interesting idea to address the suicide rate among veterans. If the Japanese could instill suicidal discipline in their troops during World War II, perhaps we could do the opposite. For example, the Ranger ethos of "I will never leave a fallen comrade behind" could be developed further to include the following: "My country needs me. I will never take my own life."

———

The fields of psychiatry and psychology have catalogued both general protective and risk factors for suicide. Protective factors include feeling loved and accepted, having strong reasons for living, including a purpose in life, and maintaining regular social engagement with others.

Unfortunately, the list of general risk factors for suicide is a long one:

- Depression
- Hopelessness
- Social alienation and isolation
- Loneliness

- Anxiety
- Chronic pain
- Sleep deprivation
- Impulsivity
- Loss of job or important relationship (e.g., divorce, break up)
- Grief
- Rage
- Guilt and shame
- Alcohol abuse
- Childhood trauma
- Perceived sense of being a burden to others
- Deteriorating cognitive health
- Employment problems
- Financial problems
- History of violence
- History of prior suicide attempts
- Family history of suicide
- Access to lethal means

Obviously, operators can check a lot of these. I've long been of the opinion that governmental "suicide prevention" efforts, suicide hotlines, platitudes about "resilience," and the VA's tone-deaf favorite—reducing access to firearms—are virtually worthless. If I'm suicidal and I call a doctor, that pre-recorded message telling me to "call 911 or go to the nearest emergency room" is probably not going to be of much use to me. (But it will probably protect the doctor, clinic, or hospital from liability.)

My view is that suicide is often an impulsive act and also an outcome that is far downstream from its root causes. The purpose of this book is to help operators find solutions to the injuries, suffering, and problems they face. I believe that with the right interventions there will be fewer suicides. Treatment really can make a massive difference in the quality of your life.

The SOF community also has the ability to help care for itself. Stay in touch with your buddies, check on them from time to time, and follow up more than once if you are worried. It is okay to ask someone quite directly if they are suicidal; you won't put the idea into their head. Make a list of reasons to live and create a plan to make it through the day, and the next day. Help your buddy problem-solve about what types of treatment he might need. Develop a concrete course of action, prioritize necessary steps, and do your best to check on him to ensure he is following through.

If you're in a dark place yourself—or what Derek Nadalini calls the "flywheel of madness"—please seek treatment, call a buddy, get sober, eat a ham sandwich (protein, carbs, fats), move your body. Don't pick up that Glock. Suicidal thoughts are usually transitory, so take a twenty-four-hour pause. Whatever pain you are in, you can stand it for one more day. Most people will feel much better within a few hours or days—and usually they are more glad than not to still be alive.

Further Recommended Readings

- *Why People Die by Suicide* by Thomas Joiner (Harvard University Press, 2007)

PART THREE

HEALING, RECOVERY, AND PERFORMANCE

CHAPTER 20

PUTTING IT ALL TOGETHER

"I took the position as Chief of Health to help address the problems my community faced. I knew we had problems. However, the injuries and impairments are even more widespread and more severe than I had imagined. No one should have to live in pain or in mental strife after years of serving their country as my brothers have. Fortunately, there are treatments and solutions that can make a profound difference."

—**Joey Fio**, former U.S. Navy SEAL, chief of health at the SEAL Future Foundation

"Healing injuries and rewiring the nervous system take time and 'the whole kitchen sink' approach. In addition to medical treatments, this includes doing the simple things like working with a counselor, regular movement in nature, journaling, breathwork, mitigating stress, avoiding or minimizing alcohol, etc."

—**Kate Pate**, neurophysiology PhD

"Reading 'Operator Syndrome' [the medical paper] took the guesswork out of the behaviors and challenges we both faced in healing

and gave me hope that with this new understanding we can tackle each challenge with compassion, understanding, diligence, and forgiveness."

—**Jen Satterly**, U.S. Army Special Forces spouse, CEO and cofounder of All Secure Foundation

"Ibogaine, an African psychedelic which has neuroregenerative properties, is a powerful therapeutic for special operators. We see impressive results when we use it to treat mTBI, PTSD, depression, and addictions. Because it has neuroregenerative properties, we have consistently seen improvements in cognition, learning, and memory. The therapeutic effect is derived from the physiological and psycho-emotional properties as well as the mystical experiences induced that greatly broaden perspective and enable a reworking of traumatizing memories. The induced altered states allow for the release of troubling emotions, as well as any sense of personal responsibility that has cemented the trauma."

—**Martin Polanco**, MD, founder and research director of The Mission Within

By now I've loaded you (perhaps overloaded you) with information about Operator Syndrome. I've described the complex and interrelated medical, psychological, existential, and interpersonal conditions and impairments that are common in the military special operations community. It's important to remember these are the result of an extremely high allostatic load, which is the accumulated weight of physiological, neurological, and neuroendocrine responses. In other words, these are quite literally physiological injuries—at the molecular and cellular level—sustained over the course of an operator's military career.

If Part Two of this book was the "bad news," then Part Three is the "good news." In this section, we have finally arrived at the solutions and treatments that can transform health, wellness, functioning, and quality of life. This current chapter describes a general approach to identify and sequence the assessments and treatments that are needed. The next chapter will provide more specific information—brief overviews—for each of the various forms of treatment that may be relevant. At the end of this chapter is a generic treatment plan for operators.

———

Be mindful that the best treatment approach for you—the operator—will be to work with a multidisciplinary medical team in the fields of neurology, psychology, psychiatry, social work, internal medicine, sleep medicine, physical therapy, endocrinology, pain management, orthopedics, regenerative medicine, etc. Ideally, this team would work together as a team, communicating directly with each other to evaluate and address all of your difficulties simultaneously. There would be a care coordinator to help you navigate your assessments and treatments, someone who would help update the treatment team with the "bouncing the ball" of your care. Moreover, this clinical team would have a very strong, nuanced, contextual understanding of what it means to be an operator or to be married to one.

Got that? Right.

Unfortunately, as you probably suspect or know, there simply aren't many programs like this, and the ones that do exist are highly flawed. This means that, for now, you have to steer most of your medical and psychological care alone. But don't be disheartened. This is quite doable for most.

One last thing: For a quick review of Operator Syndrome, you can read our original medical paper, and you can share it with others. Don't be intimidated, for while this paper is published in a medical journal, it was actually written for you, in a format and at a level that most folks should be able to read and understand. Also, you can use this paper to help educate your medical providers on the breadth and nature of your injuries.

———

The aim of this chapter is to provide an understanding of the necessary comprehensive and multidisciplinary approach required, the importance of having a partner in the process, the obstacles you are likely to face, and—most importantly—a recommended general sequence of assessments and treatments to help guide you. Please understand this is a very general strategy for approaching your care, but each operator will need to make their own individual adjustments as necessary.

We have to start with suicide risk assessment. This is mission-critical. Are you suicidal? Does someone you trust think you are suicidal? If so, please seek immediate medical attention.

Next, let's consider what you need to do for preparation.

First, you must have honest conversations—with yourself, your partner, your friends, and others you trust. You can complete the one-page Operator Syndrome Scale included in this book. This is a short self-report questionnaire that can be completed quickly. It is not a diagnostic instrument per se, but it can help give you a quick snapshot of the conditions and problems you may wish to seek help for. You can also bring it to your primary care appointment. It can even be a tool to track your progress over time, perhaps at three- or six-month intervals.

Next, you really need to have a primary care provider (PCP). If you don't have one, find one. A PCP is usually an MD or osteopathic doctor (either family medicine or internal medicine) but can also be a physician's assistant or advance practice nurse. They are generalists and function as the "gate-keepers" to virtually all medical care. They are the ones that conduct general physical exams, order blood lab tests, make referrals to all specialists, and help manage your ongoing care. PCPs are the quarterbacks of modern healthcare.

Be aware that a comprehensive, multidisciplinary ap-proach is necessary. I call this the "whole systems approach" because its perspective takes into account every relevant sys-tem. Obviously, this heavily encompasses your biological sys-tems (e.g., central and peripheral nervous, circulatory, gastro-intestinal, respiratory, endocrine, perceptual, musculoskeletal) as well as psychological and cognitive functioning. It also en-compasses family and social systems around you, including whom you live with, work for, socialize with, and engage with in your community.

It will really help you to enlist a partner you trust and who knows you well throughout this process. A spouse or long-term romantic partner will be best for most operators. You can also, and probably should, recruit a buddy or two—as in a "swim buddy," "battle buddy," or "fire team buddy." You will benefit from this support and encouragement. A partner can hold you accountable and also be someone to help problem-solve or call you when things become difficult (which they will). Let's face it: when it comes to health and healthcare, stoic men almost always do better if their wife or another partner is supporting them.

Finally, be aware that you will face many logistical and funding challenges due to the nature of modern medicine and how we pay for it. Do not let that thwart you. Be assertive with your medical providers and insist on what you need. If what you need for care is not supported by the VA healthcare system or insurance providers, call around to some of the SOF foundations. Many of them can make specific referral suggestions and offer financial support for treatments (e.g., hyperbaric oxygen therapy) that might not otherwise be available to you.

––––––––––

I wish there were more high-quality, comprehensive, specialty treatment programs for operators. Unfortunately, right now there are very few. That means you have to take an assertive, proactive approach to seek and find the care you need. You already know there are many obstacles standing in the way of your recovery, but I'll list them again anyway, because being forewarned is being forearmed:

- Civilian society does not understand what operators experienced or did, or the personal cost of their service.
- Healthcare providers, medical systems, and bureaucracies are generally preoccupied with "social justice" and are hostile to the notion that operators require specialty care models and treatments to treat their unique injuries.

- Within the VA and in modern medicine, there is a tendency to diagnose (often misdiagnose) veterans with PTSD, while ignoring other injuries and medical needs.
- There is a genuine lack of medical and scientific knowledge on how to treat TBI, hormonal dysfunction, sleep disorders, chronic pain, addiction, etc.
- There are massive systemic gaps and fragmentation of care in modern medicine—for example, your therapist is unlikely to ever speak with your endocrinologist.
- The limitations of insurance and funding models are unlikely to cover the costs of many powerful treatments, especially novel interventions that are not currently in the mainstream of medical care (e.g., hyperbaric oxygen, ketamine infusion therapy, hot sauna, psychedelic medicines, etc.).
- There are few medical providers—even in the DOD—who have any contextualized understanding of who operators are, what they have done and been exposed to, and what their needs are.

Your recovery will necessarily require you to be assertive and persistent in the face of disappointments and frustrations. It will involve some trial and error to find what works for you. It may include interventions that are considered "alternative" or "complementary" by the medical establishment. And it *must* involve a focus on lifestyle and habits, including your sleep, diet, exercise, social relationships, and pursuit of meaning in life.

Perhaps the best single piece of advice I can give you now is to approach your recovery like you did your career in special operations: never quit, never give up.

What follows is a recommended approach—where to start and how to sequence assessments and interventions. This is intended to help *guide* you in your healing and recovery. Remember, this is only a very general strategy. It is *not* a specific treatment program, and it does not indicate specific treatments for any one individual. You will have to work to develop a treatment program that is specific to your needs and priorities, and you will need to make decisions and adjustments as you go. At the end of this chapter is an example treatment plan that you may refer to, modifying it as necessary—hopefully in collaboration with your PCP and partner.

Ready? Let's get to it.

Step 1: Are you suicidal? Does someone you trust think you are suicidal? If so, please seek immediate medical attention.

Step 2: Have honest conversations—with yourself, your wife or partner, and others you trust. Review the Operator Syndrome Scale, maybe even complete it for yourself. You should also enlist your wife or a partner to accompany you, coax you, encourage you, and help you keep track of things. Consider reaching out to relevant beneficent foundations for guidance. Review your lifestyle and daily habits. Consider areas for improvement, such as sleep, substance use, diet, exercise, relaxation, relationships, hobbies, recovery practices, etc. (see Chapter 23).

Step 3: Do you have a PCP? If not, get one ASAP and schedule an appointment.

Step 4: Attend your primary care appointment. Bring the Operator Syndrome paper and discuss. You will probably have to help educate your PCP. Get a general medical evaluation.

Unless clearly unnecessary, request the following evaluations:

- Blood lab tests of metabolic functioning
- Blood lab tests of endocrine (hormone) functioning, especially testosterone
- Testing for heavy metals
- Testing for parasites specific to your deployment areas of operation
- A polysomnography ("sleep study")
- Psychiatric and psychological assessments
- Orthopedic, chiropractic, and physical therapy assessments for mobility and chronic pain management
- Neurological assessments for TBI, cognitive functioning, and headaches or migraines

Step 5: Keep all scheduled appointments and follow-up care. Identify all relevant clinical targets. Ask yourself: "At this point, is there anything urgent that I have not yet addressed and that cannot wait?" If possible, consider trying to identify a comprehensive, immersive treatment program that might be appropriate for you.

Step 6: Begin the treatments prescribed or recommended by your providers. The next chapter provides a brief explanation for many of the treatments you may benefit from. Also, see the example treatment plan at the end of this chapter. Common treatments are likely to include:

- Stellate ganglion block therapy (preferably bilateral, in most cases)
- Ketamine infusion therapy
- Cognitive behavioral psychotherapy

- Couples counseling to educate spouse, reduce conflict, and increase relationship satisfaction
- Pain management (non-pharmacological), or physical therapy
- Headache and migraine treatment
- Psychiatric medications (*always optional*)
- Sleep hygiene therapy (i.e., cognitive behavioral therapy, or iCBT)
- Addiction treatment
- Vestibular therapy (for symptoms of disequilibrium and vertigo)
- Speech pathology (to improve cognitive functioning)
- Transcranial magnetic stimulation (specifically the MeRT variation)
- Hyperbaric oxygen therapy
- Treatments for vision and hearing problems
- Regenerative medicine treatments
- Psychedelic plant medicines

Step 7: Follow an anti-inflammatory diet and develop lifestyle habits that support brain health and psychological functioning (see Chapter 23). This involves the following:

- Minimize or eliminate consumption of soda, fast food, junk food, added sugars, highly processed foods (e.g., most frozen dinners, canned soups).
- Eat a whole food diet (e.g., Mediterranean Diet or DASH), high in quality protein.
- Consider dietary supplementation with omega-3, vitamin D, turmeric, and B vitamins.
- Consider intermittent fasting.

- Minimize or eliminate use of alcohol and tobacco.
- Exercise regularly and moderately (e.g., walking, variable-resistance band strength training).
- Improve the quality of sleep by following natural sleep hygiene methods such as environmental engineering of your bedroom (e.g., keeping it dark, cool, quiet, and comfortable).
- Use daily recovery practices known to reduce chronic systemic inflammation (e.g., hot sauna bathing, cold immersion, meditation, yoga, stretching, prayer, time in nature, float therapy, or hobbies).

Step 8: Consider any transition processes and services that you might need.

———————

AAR. Make necessary adjustments. Keep going.

Example of a Specific Operator Syndrome Treatment Plan

Scheduling of primary care appointment to review general medical health in the context of Operator Syndrome, receive referrals to necessary interventions, and coordinate care. It is suggested to bring this book or the original Operator Syndrome medical paper with you to educate your medical provider.

1. Laboratory blood panels to evaluate hormonal functioning (e.g., testosterone, thyroid, estrogen, HGH). Hormonal abnormalities are common in people with extensive blast exposures and TBI.
2. Testing for metabolic functioning (typically part of a basic physical exam)

3. Testing for heavy metals

4. Testing for parasites

5. Polysomnography (sleep study) and sleep medicine consultation to evaluate for sleep disorders, including obstructive sleep apnea and periodic limb movement disorder

6. Stellate ganglion block therapy (or cervical sympathetic blockade), preferably a bilateral course

7. Ketamine infusion therapy, which may be synergistic with stellate ganglion block therapy

8. Cognitive behavioral psychotherapy. Individual psychotherapy is recommended for one to two sessions per week for at least three to six months, and possibly "booster" sessions on occasion after that.

9. Couples counseling to educate spouse, reduce conflict, enrich intimacy, and increase marital satisfaction

10. Pain management consultation and treatment (non-pharmacological)

11. Headache and migraine consultation and treatment

12. Possible use of psychiatric medications, such as antidepressants (e.g., SSRIs) and mood stabilizers (e.g., lamotrigine to help reduce rage)

13. Sleep hygiene therapy (i.e., iCBT), a specific form of cognitive behavioral therapy to improve sleep. Six to twelve iCBT therapy sessions are recommended.

14. Neuropsychological cognitive testing, brain neuroimaging, and neurological assessment to better understand cognitive deficits and brain health

15. Reduction or elimination of alcohol, recreational drugs, or tobacco use, if relevant

16. Anti-inflammatory diet and lifestyle habits, important for supporting brain health and psychological functioning. This involves doing the following:
    a. Minimize or eliminate consumption of soda, fast food, junk food, added sugars, highly processed foods (e.g., most frozen dinners and canned soups).
    b. Eat a whole food diet (e.g., Mediterranean or DASH diets), high in quality protein.
    c. Consider dietary supplementation with omega-3, vitamin D, turmeric, and B vitamins.
    d. Consider intermittent fasting.
    e. Minimize or eliminate use of alcohol and tobacco.
    f. Exercise regularly and moderately (e.g., walking, variable-resistance band strength training).
    g. Improve the quality of your sleep by following natural sleep hygiene methods such as environmental engineering of your bedroom (e.g., keeping it dark, cool, quiet, and comfortable).
    h. Use daily recovery practices known to reduce chronic systemic inflammation (e.g., hot sauna bathing, cold immersion, meditation, yoga, prayer, or time in nature).
17. Consider comprehensive rehabilitation for TBI at an intensive outpatient program (e.g., Marcus Brain Institute, Shepardsmen, THRIVE program, or HomeBase).
18. Consider other treatments, including speech pathology, transcranial magnetic stimulation (specifically the MeRT variation), hyperbaric oxygen therapy, regenerative medicine approaches, vestibular therapy, other psychedelic plant medicines.

CHAPTER 21

THE INTERVENTIONS

"One of the most challenging things—and I still struggle with this—is to ask for help. Then again, if I wanted to learn a new weapon system or tactic, I asked for help. I'm the wisest when I allow others to help me and get out of my own way."
—**Herb Thompson**, U.S. Army Special Forces 5th Group Team Sergeant (Ret.), author of *The Transition Mission*

"I interviewed over seventy-five current and former Navy SEALs for my doctoral scholarship. Of those, at least seventy of them reported community-wide, reiterative symptoms, including an inability to recover from routine training evolutions, insomnia and interrupted sleep, unexplained chronic pain, severe trauma symptoms (that didn't meet diagnostic criteria of PTSD), rumination, impaired cognition and attention, and adverse interpersonal relationship patterns. Operator Syndrome is now the conceptual framework of my practice with all Special Operators. It's where we start."
—**Rebecca Ann Ivory**, DNP, board-certified psychiatric-mental health nurse practitioner, MS, at the Washington School of Nursing

"Whatever you'd like to call it that I was experiencing, whatever parts of my past life created it (childhood, contact sports from seven years old, football through college, breaching, multiple head traumas, war, transition, etc.), it was present and deteriorating. Psychedelic medicine reset me."

—**Marcus Capone**, U.S. Navy SEAL (Ret.),
cofounder of VETS Inc., cofounder of TARA Mind

"Operator Syndrome (OS) summarized is what really happens to our special operation forces personnel. It is essential to recognize and acknowledge with patients that they are not going 'crazy,' that OS is a real physiological condition. It must be addressed biologically as well as psychologically. I have developed a highly effective treatment protocol using ketamine (to regrow brain tissue) and stellate ganglion block to reduce PTSD and anxiety symptoms caused by an overactive sympathetic nervous system. We CAN treat this syndrome!"

—**Eugene Lipov**, MD, coauthor of *The Invisible Machine: The Startling Truth about Trauma and the Scientific Breakthrough That Can Transform Your Life*

"Try it all and see what is most beneficial for your well-being and your family. What I have noticed on my journey is different things work for different people."

—**Daniel Luna**, EdD, U.S. Navy SEAL (Ret.)

As I have said several times already by now, Operator Syndrome conditions are highly treatable. The purpose of this chapter is to list, define, and explain some of the powerful therapies that can turn an operator's life around and restore health, functioning, relationships, and quality of life. Traditional mental healthcare interventions (therapy, psychiatric medications, etc.) are the most widely used treatments for PTSD and depression in Western medicine. I will begin with a short primer on them. However, there are also *many* other effective treatments available. Some of these interventions even seem to trigger the growth of new neurons and dendrites, as well as strengthen and develop pathways and connections within the brain; that is, they may directly treat TBI at the neuronal level.

———————

Traditional mental healthcare typically involves two components: psychotherapy and psychiatric medications. Each may be used by itself, but they are commonly recommended to be used together, at least in the initial phases of treating a recently diagnosed psychiatric disorder.

Psychotherapy

"At my Center, we know that post-traumatic stress is multidimensional in nature and that treatment must be comprehensive in scope and use cutting-edge technologies. Our treatment program uses virtual reality to enhance standard exposure therapy, and we add a group component to directly target anger, depression, sleep, and moral injury. Also, rather than sessions once a week or once a month, we offer an intensive outpatient program (IOP) that provides this comprehensive approach in a three-week program, with results that are two to three times better than standard PTSD treatment programs."

—**Deborah C. Beidel**, PhD, professor of psychology, director of UCF RESTORES at University of Central Florida

Talking to a professionally trained therapist can be a powerful change agent. Often referred to as "counseling" or "therapy," this kind of treatment has many different orientations, including cognitive-behavioral, interpersonal, humanistic, psychodynamic, and others. Most therapists are somewhat eclectic in their practice, using ideas and approaches from more than one school of thought. The good news is that any talking therapy that focuses on emotions, thoughts, or behaviors can help alleviate psychological distress and lead to remission or even a longstanding cure for psychiatric disorders. Therapy may be conducted in an individual, couples, or group format. Some therapies are time-limited and highly structured, with workbooks and weekly homework assignments.

Cognitive-behavioral therapy (CBT) arguably has the strongest research base of support. This approach focuses on changing maladaptive thoughts and behavioral habits in order to treat depression, anxiety, PTSD, anger, insomnia, chronic pain, borderline personality disorder, and addictions. It also helps with management of chronic diseases (e.g., diabetes) and weight loss.

Within the broad category of CBT, there are general approaches and also specifically branded interventions. Exposure therapy or counterconditioning involves exposing people to the memories or objects that elicit anxiety and distress. It works through the principles of habituation and extinction and is probably the most effective form of therapy to treat PTSD.

For a person with a snake phobia, we would literally expose them to snakes (safely) via photos, videos, and perhaps, eventually, live animals. Over the course of six to twelve sessions, especially if supplemented with snake-themed homework assignments, the fear of snakes will fade away. Another more common example is the fear of public speaking, which can often be treated through CBT by having the person give talks—first to themselves, then to their therapist, and then to other people. (Toastmasters provides this for free, combining the exposure of giving talks with regular practice and coaching—all classic elements of CBT.)

Treating the fear-reactivity symptoms of PTSD from combat, sexual assault, or interpersonal violence is obviously a little more complicated than treating phobic reactions to snakes. But the principles are the same. We expose people to memories of their traumatic experiences. To do this we use their imagination to recreate the traumatic experience over and over again, as vividly as possible. Some programs even use virtual reality to enhance the exposure intensity, engaging all of the senses: sights, sounds, odors, even vibrations through programming such as Virtual Iraq.

Exposure therapy usually takes two or three sessions a week, for a total of twelve to sixteen total sessions, so it is efficient. In addition, there is usually homework between sessions. Examples of assignments might include listening to audiotapes of the exposure sessions, keeping a journal, and undergoing "real life" activities that might otherwise be avoided—such as visiting a grave, looking at unit photos, calling an old buddy, etc.

Within the category of exposure therapy there are three branded treatments: cognitive processing therapy (CPT), prolonged exposure (PE), and eye movement desensitization and reprocessing (EMDR). Each of these works mostly by using a specific method for applying the exposure to traumatic memories. Somewhat outside the exposure therapies, is another branded CBT treatment called dialectical behavior therapy (DBT). Initially developed as a treatment for borderline personality disorder, DBT is a smorgasbord of different types of activities and conversations. In addition to treating personality disorders, it is also quite effective in helping people learn to manage chronic rage and suicidality. All of these treatments are usually available through the VA healthcare system, as well as from private-sector therapists.

Therapists can come from a variety of training backgrounds. They may be psychologists (PhD, PsyD, MA), social workers (MSW), nurses (DNP, ARNP), and psychiatrists (MD). In recent years, I've also seen impressive work by many of the veterans' programs using peer-to-peer support counseling. The challenge is finding a counselor you can feel comfortable with, and let's face it: not many therapists, even those who work for the VA, have much understanding of operators or other combatants, particularly the challenges they face in civilian life. Unfortunately, this is more true than ever as mental health training programs have placed increasing emphasis on social justice activism—even within the context of treating individuals for severe psychiatric disorders. Just remember, if your therapist is not a good fit for you, you always have the right to find a different therapist.

Psychiatric Medications

Psychiatrists (MDs with residency specialty training) used to receive considerable training in psychotherapy, primarily Freudian psychoanalysis. However, as more and more pharmaceuticals came to market, they shifted their focus to prescribing and managing psychiatric medications. If there was a clear tipping point at any moment in time, it was probably 1987, when Prozac came to market. Very few psychiatrists now provide any traditional psychotherapy at all.

Today we now have a large number of different psychiatric medications to address a diverse range of symptoms. While newer medications are perhaps a little better than their psychiatric predecessors from the 1950s to the '80s, I don't believe the overall impact of psychiatric medications for any given individual is really all that different. Modern "atypical" antipsychotics are a considerable step up from older antipsychotics in terms of a less severe side effect profile, but the difference is relative. "Atypicals" still cause weight gain and metabolic syndromes, including diabetes.

Psychiatric medications can be divided into a number of categories based on mechanisms of action (e.g., SSRIs, benzodiazepines), or they can be sorted by purpose. Most of these medications are intended to be taken daily, with only a few that may be used on an "as needed" basis. An antidepressant won't help if you only take it on the days that you feel especially down—it needs to be taken every day in order to have the intended antidepressant effect. Also, be mindful that most medications have both a generic or scientific name and at least one brand name (e.g., fluoxetine = Prozac). This can be a source of confusion.

The following sections describe some of the most commonly prescribed medications for operators.

Antidepressants

Older antidepressants (e.g., amitriptyline, trazodone) are still around, but they are rarely prescribed for depression anymore. Instead, medications in the family of selective serotonin reuptake inhibitors[9] (SSRIs) are most commonly used. There are at least six different SSRIs, including Lexapro, Celexa, Prozac,

---

9   The name is a description of the mechanism of action. These medications facilitate the transmission of the neurotransmitter serotonin.

Paxil, Zoloft, and Pexeva. There are also other forms of newer antidepressants. Serotonin and norepinephrine reuptake inhibitors (SNRIs) include Effexor, Cymbalta, Pristiq, and others. Although often prescribed for depression, the medication bupropion (brand name Wellbutrin) does not fit into either of the two major antidepressant categories. Bupropion is also used to help with smoking cessation (usually under the brand name Zyban).

Antidepressants are the most commonly prescribed psychiatric medications and one of the most widely prescribed form of any type of medication. They often have side effects of nausea, headaches, agitation, weight gain, and problems with sexual functioning. These side effects are most prominent early in the course of treatment and often subside after four to twelve weeks, but it is usually wise to start with a low dose and increase slowly over time. For a twenty-milligram prescription of Lexapro, for example, one might start with five milligrams per day for a week, then ten milligrams per day for a week or two, etc. This allows the body to adjust gradually.

While antidepressants do not cause a "high" and are not addictive in the formal sense of the word, they can cause "discontinuation" effects if ceased abruptly in about 15 to 25 percent of people. SSRI discontinuation can feel like flu symptoms; it can also temporarily impair concentration or create an odd sensory experience sometimes referred to as "brain zaps." If stopping an antidepressant, it is best to do it gradually and under medical supervision.

How effective are antidepressants? For some people, they are game changers; for others their effects are modest—or negligible. The reasons for this uncertainty are twofold. First, we don't have an easy way to know which one of the many antidepressants will work for any given individual. A process of trial and error is common, and many people go through two to four medications before they find one that works for them, or they give up. Assume any given antidepressant has a 25 to 45 percent chance of working for you. Pharmacogenetic testing can help narrow the list of likely effective antidepressants, but insurance programs generally will not pay for this service, and most prescribers do not know how to use it. The second reason involves lag times. Because antidepressants have a long half-life (meaning they stay in your body for a long time), it usually takes six to twelve weeks before enough medication has accumulated in the body to represent a therapeutic dose. Once the right drug and dosage are found, however, antidepressants can be reasonably helpful at reducing symptoms of depression and anxiety.

Sleep Aids

In the early 1990s at the start of my career, the most common sleep aids prescribed by my psychiatrist colleagues at the VA were trazodone (an older antidepressant) and diphenhydramine (a.k.a. Benadryl). And yes, over-the-counter antihistamines are also reasonably effective for most people. In addition, a class of sleep aids known as "hypnotics" (e.g., Ambien, Lunesta) came on the market in the early 1990s.

Thanks to heavy advertising and a concerted push by pharmaceutical reps inside hospitals, hypnotics seem to have replaced trazodone and diphenhydramine as the sleep aids of choice for many prescribers. However, hypnotics have significant potential for side effects, including a "hangover" effect and very active sleepwalking episodes. I had patients who drove to a store or cooked and ate meals in their sleep. One patient shaved off his beard in the middle of the night. He practically jumped out of his skin the next morning when he looked in the mirror.

None of these sleep aids are really very good for our sleep, especially on a long-term basis. They may help increase sleep quantity in the short term, but they also disrupt the quality of sleep by altering the time we spend in REM or slow-wave sleep. They have a place to help with sleep in the very short term (between two and five days) and with intermittent use, but it is usually not advisable to use them every night for any length of time.

There are two other medications for sleep that you should be aware of. A nightly *low* dose of gabapentin can help improve sleep by reducing periodic limb movements during the night, and it may be taken indefinitely without much in the way of side effects. Another medication named Prazosin, a medication for high blood pressure, has been widely used off-label to help reduce nightmares in people with PTSD. Some operators have found it to be somewhat helpful.

Stimulants

Stimulant medications such as Adderall, Ritalin, and Vyvanse are used to treat attention-deficit hyperactivity disorder (ADHD). Because they improve concentration and increase energy, they are often sought as a performance enhancer by people who do not have ADHD. They can be addictive and also may raise blood pressure and heart rate, increasing blood sugar. Be careful.

Antianxiety Medications

There are dozens of drugs in the family of benzodiazepines (most commonly Librium, Valium, Ativan, Xanax, Klonopin), which slow the activity of the central nervous system. Prior to the advent of Prozac in 1987, they were the most commonly prescribed class of drug in the world. They have the effect of sedating, reducing anxiety, and relaxing muscles. Currently they are an important medication to help reduce the symptoms of alcohol withdrawal. However, they are no longer recommended for treating PTSD or anxiety disorders because they are extremely addicting. Not only do people build up tolerance quickly, but they can have adverse effects on cognition, memory, balance, and judgment. They also have a strong, dangerous interaction with alcohol, and it is possible to overdose. Be very careful.

Beta blockers (e.g., propranolol), used to treat hypertension, are sometimes prescribed to reduce anxiety, especially on an as-needed basis in situations that provoke excessive fear (e.g., flying, public speaking). They can reduce many of the physiological symptoms of anxiety without producing a "high" or interfering with cognitive functioning or judgment.

Mood Stabilizers

Medications that help control mood swings between depression and mania are known as mood stabilizers. Lithium, for example, is a heavy metal and the primary treatment for bipolar disorder. Lamotrigine may be prescribed as a secondary medicine for bipolar disorder, but it is also effective in reducing agitation, rage, and explosive anger outbursts. Anticonvulsant medications (e.g., gabapentin, topiramate) may also be used off-label as mood stabilizers.

Antipsychotics

Medications such as Risperdal, Seroquel, Zyprexa, Clozaril, Haldol, and Abilify are prescribed to reduce delusions, hallucinations, and paranoid thoughts. In addition to treating schizophrenia, they are also sometimes used as a secondary medication for bipolar disorder. While fairly effective at reducing psychotic symptoms, they also involve very serious side effects of weight gain, diabetes, cardiovascular problems, agitation, apathy, abnormal movements, and many more. Be very, very careful.

Addiction Medications

Unfortunately, we don't really have very good medications to treat substance abuse. Benzodiazepines are used effectively to prevent symptoms of alcohol withdrawal, but they are highly addictive themselves, so they are only used for several days at a time during a medical detoxification. Low dose bupropion is prescribed to help with cigarette smoking cessation. Naltrexone, an opioid antagonist, can be useful for reducing alcohol cravings and minimizing alcohol use—but only after a heavy drinker has already detoxed or cut way down. Other medications, such as gabapentin and topiramate, might be prescribed to help manage irritability and anxiety symptoms that often appear after several weeks of sobriety.

Some of these psychiatric medications may be appropriate and helpful, but you must also remember that taking prescription medications is never a requirement—it is always optional.

Although mental healthcare interventions involving therapy and medications are the most common treatments for psychiatric disorders, there are also *many* other treatments available. Furthermore, many of the conditions in Operator Syndrome are not psychiatric disorders per se. What follows are short, alphabetically arranged descriptions of other interventions commonly used by operators. Be aware that some of these treatments do not currently have full medical research to support them as treatments for the conditions they are often used for (e.g., some psychedelic compounds).

Addiction Treatments

There are many treatment options for alcohol and drug abuse disorders. These include outpatient individual therapy, group counseling, medications (e.g., naltrexone for alcohol cravings), peer support programs (e.g., Alcoholics Anonymous), detoxification units, and residential sobriety programs. See Chapter 11 for more information on addiction treatment.

Cognitive Rehabilitation Therapy (CRT)

Cognitive rehabilitation therapy is used to improve cognitive functioning after a brain injury, stroke, brain tumor removal, or other brain disorder. A form of therapy, it can help develop new cognitive skills and strategies in order to compensate for cognitive impairments.

Continuous Positive Airway Pressure (CPAP) Machine

The most common treatment for obstructive sleep apnea is a CPAP machine, which works by pushing air to the upper respiratory tract at a constant pressure via a tube and mask worn over the nose (and sometimes mouth) during sleep, allowing the airways to remain open and unobstructed.

Couples Counseling

Marital or couples counseling is a specialized form of therapy, usually involving one therapist working with a romantically involved couple. It can be used to improve communication, reduce conflict, align expectations, reconcile major differences, and enhance sexual intimacy, in order to preserve or enrich the relationship. In truth, couples counseling is frequently used covertly to help one partner ease into a breakup gently, hoping to maintain an amiable relationship after separation. Maintaining a cooperative relationship after a breakup is especially important if the couple share young children. I often recommend a few sessions of couples counseling to operators as a way to educate their partners about Operator Syndrome and develop a collaborative effort toward better health.

Hormonal Therapies

"The source of endocrine dysfunction isn't always obvious. To optimize the operator's health and functioning it is therefore imperative to identify the source. For example, poor sleep will down-regulate testosterone production, but low testosterone production commonly leads to poor sleep. Simply replacing low hormones is oftentimes not likely to be the optimal approach in treating endocrine issues. The operator will always be better served and be more resilient if he is able to produce and regulate his endogenous hormones naturally."

—**Kirk Parsley**, MD, former U.S. Navy SEAL,
physician to the SEALs

"The endocrine system is the canary in the mine shaft. The body knows when to shut down unnecessary activities (such as reproduction) when you are under profound physical stress. If the canary dies, you can get another one, but the miners will still succumb to gas poisoning. It is important to determine if a hormone abnormality is a primary endocrine disease that is not likely to change, or a secondary and potentially reversible response to other

factors, which operators are prone to experience. Charlatans prey on people with complex medical conditions, and hormone-related scams are everywhere. Make sure you see a qualified practitioner who orders testing in a legitimate laboratory and does not invent diseases for profit. Temporary hormone supplementation is okay, but take the long view of what will allow your endocrine system to function optimally on its own."

—**Richard Auchus**, MD, PhD, former U.S. Air
Force Medical Corps endocrinologist, professor
of pharmacology and internal medicine at the
University of Michigan

As described in Chapter 4, most operators experience a drop in testosterone production after a period of extensive blast wave exposures, high op tempos, sleep deprivation, and other brain injuries. Many also experience abnormalities in thyroid, cortisol, estrogen, and human growth hormone. Each of these hormonal imbalances might require different evaluations, and some might indicate a need for interventions.

A first step is to get appropriate screening blood tests to evaluate each hormone system. The tests should be ordered and interpreted by a qualified practitioner using a certified laboratory with validated tests and normal ranges. You might be instructed to have some tests drawn at a particular time of day, with or without fasting. Borderline tests might require further dynamic testing designed to stimulate or suppress the hormone in question. Just because a laboratory test is outside the normal range does not necessarily mean that a disease is present, that treatment is required, or that the condition is permanent.

Low testosterone production may be treated by adding exogenous testosterone to the body via creams, shots, or pellets.

However, testosterone replacement therapy (TRT) is usually *not* the preferred place to start, because TRT will suppress the body's ability to subsequently produce your own testosterone, and it might cause infertility or other significant side effects. Other, less risk-prone interventions may be effective at helping the body naturally raise its testosterone production. Dietary changes, nutritional supplements (e.g., zinc), good sleep quality, avoidance of certain medications, and recovery practices can provide substantial improvements to testosterone levels in men. For other hormone deficiencies or excess, specific medications may be necessary after the diagnosis is established.[10]

Hyperbaric Oxygen Therapy (HBOT)

HBOT involves sitting in a dive chamber while pure oxygen is delivered at a higher-than-normal atmospheric pressure. The treatment is usually thirty to forty sessions, and each session lasts for sixty to 120 minutes. Although medical studies have not shown conclusively that HBOT is an effective treatment for TBI, there is some evidence it could be a game changer for many. Anecdotally, it is very common among operators to have tried this intervention, and I know many guys who report profound benefits in cognition, balance, and headaches. Because there is wide variation in the nature of TBIs, it seems intuitive that the same treatment will not work the same for everyone with a TBI.

Ketamine Infusion

Ketamine therapy has FDA approval for the treatment of depression. It involves infusions of ketamine delivered intravenously in low doses over four to eight outpatient sessions. The reason for the extended period is that the drug's antidepressant

---

10   Special thanks to Richard Auchus, MD, PhD, for his mentorship and help with this section.

effects tend to become more prolonged with repeated exposure. Ketamine therapy generally includes a psychotherapeutic intervention that allows the patient to explore and discuss their experience with a mental health professional who can help identify positive thoughts, feelings, and realizations, with the goal of helping them retain positive changes in beliefs, attitudes, and perspectives. Some of us believe that ketamine may amplify benefits of stellate ganglion block therapy, ease existential concerns, relieve anxiety or PTSD symptoms, and promote neural plasticity. I do not recommend using ketamine tablets or other forms of delivery at this point in time.

Occupational Therapy

The goal of occupational therapy is to target problems in functioning caused by physical and mental impairments. Occupational therapists work with patients, families, and caregivers to develop methods and strategies to improve functioning in daily living, relationships, and work. For instance, occupational therapists may assist in modifying living or workspaces or provide training on assistive devices and technologies. They also work closely with other healthcare professionals to provide ongoing support, facilitate skill acquisition, and assist with life transitions.

Orthopedic Interventions: Surgery, Chiropractic, Physical Therapy

Orthopedic assessments and interventions involve medical treatments or procedures that focus on the musculoskeletal system (i.e., bones, joints, muscles, ligaments, tendons, and related structures). Common orthopedic interventions may include surgeries, physical therapy, pain management techniques, or assistive medical devices such as braces, inserts, crutches, etc.

Pain Management (Non-Pharmaceutical)

Chronic pain management includes a variety of interventions and strategies. CBT therapists aim to identify and modify maladaptive or distorted thoughts that have developed around the experience of pain and that may contribute to a heightened pain sensitivity. With this sensitivity, known as hyperalgesia, you feel pain where it is normal to, but the level of pain experienced is excessive. This can occur even after an injury is healed, when the pain receptors continue to send signals after they should have stopped doing so. CBT or behavioral medicine approaches from a specially trained therapist can help reduce this phenomenon.

Other interventions like physical therapy aim to reduce pain while increasing physical mobility and functionality. Multidisciplinary pain management programs seek to address factors contributing to pain at multiple levels (e.g., physical or medical, psychological, vocational, social, environmental). Other pain management interventions include corticosteroid injections, biofeedback, massage therapy, and other recovery modalities (e.g., meditation, yoga, stretching, cold immersion). Float tank therapy may provide special benefits by removing all compression from joints and the spine for a period of time.

Psychedelic Medicines

"Marcus's primary diagnosis of PTSD never fully made sense to me…there was so much more to what we were experiencing. He thoroughly loved his job, teammates, and deploying overseas, so when the micro-changes we'd been seeing over time became greatly exacerbated during the transition to civilian life, I felt both frantic and hopeless. Western medicine approaches had failed us, and it felt as though time was running out. As a last-ditch effort to save Marcus and our family, I arranged for him to leave the

U.S., for a treatment that seemed absolutely crazy to us: psyche-delic therapy with ibogaine and 5-MeO-DMT. We had nothing left to lose at that point, so when he emerged as the man I'd met twenty years earlier, we both knew we had to pay this healing forward to our friends and other veterans."

—**Amber Capone**, U.S. Navy SEAL spouse,
cofounder and executive director of VETS: Veterans
Exploring Treatment Solutions, Inc.

Psychedelic medicine is the therapeutic use of psychoactive substances derived from either plant compounds (e.g., psilocy-bin, ibogaine, ayahuasca, 5-MeO-DMT) or synthetically made compounds (MDMA).[11] They have been used to treat existen-tial angst, depression, PTSD, substance abuse, and aspects of pain and TBI. Many of these compounds are currently illegal in the U.S., but psilocybin and MDMA now have a pretty good body of medical research to support their effectiveness.

I expect psilocybin and MDMA will be mainstream treatments for depression and PTSD in the very near future. Research supporting the use of other psychedelics is farther be-hind but ongoing, and it will likely shape the future of mental healthcare. There are psychedelic programs in countries other than the U.S. where these other compounds are not illegal. For example, one program south of the U.S-Mexico border near San Diego provides a two-night retreat, with ibogaine used the first night and 5-MeO-DMT the second.

Psychedelics initiate a "trip" or "journey" (thirty minutes to twelve hours in length) that can bring about deep changes in mood, thoughts, perspectives, and behaviors, and *perhaps* even trigger neural plasticity. Often these treatments are accompanied

---

11   3,4-methylenedioxymethamphetamine; commonly known as "ecstasy" or "molly."

by a therapist or facilitator, and include the use of journaling, rituals, or some other "integration" practice. These are not ongoing treatments—they are more "one and done"—although some people use them once or a twice a year for several years.

Psychedelic medicines have become quite popular in the operator community, and I know many people (spouses included) who describe profound and lasting benefits across virtually every area of their life. However, be aware that we are in the very early stages of understanding these medicines. We also know there are serious risks, including blood pressure spikes or cardiac arrest, psychosis, and "bad trips" that can leave a lasting sense of distress. I recommend these treatments only be used under medical supervision. "Micro-dosing" also seems to be somewhat in vogue, but we know very little about it—and the definition itself can refer to widely different practices.

Bottom line: psychedelics have great promise, but they are not without risks, and we should learn much more about their effects before considering them for mainstream use.

Regenerative Medicine: Stem Cells, Exomes, Peptides, Orthobiologics

The goal of regenerative medicine is to repair or regenerate damaged tissue and organs by using biomedical technology and treatment techniques (e.g., stem cells, orthobiologics, peptides, exomes, and tissue engineering) to activate the body's natural reparative processes.

Sleep Hygiene and iCBT

"*The most effective modality of treatment for most sleep disorders (other than apnea) is cognitive behavioral therapy for insomnia.*"

—**Robert Sweetman**, former U.S. Navy SEAL

Sleep hygiene refers to a collection of behavioral habits and environmental engineering to promote optimal sleep quantity and quality. Good sleep hygiene means having nightly bedtime rituals that promote relaxation (e.g., putting away screens, stopping work or school-related activities prior to bedtime), and a comfortable sleeping environment (e.g., cool, dark, quiet). A special form of CBT therapy known as iCBT exists to help develop these routines and has been shown to be quite effective—and without the use of any pharmaceuticals. For more information, including specific recommendations, see Chapter 3.

Speech-Language Pathology

Speech-language pathology, also referred to as speech therapy, specializes in the assessment and treatment of communication-related disorders and impairments. Treatment can focus on improving speech (e.g., word slurring, a potential symptom of TBI), organization and planning, communication-related skills, and strategies for maintaining concentration and improving memory. Because language and cognition are inextricably linked, it can be very helpful for multiple aspects of TBI.

Stellate Ganglion Block (SGB) Therapy or Cervical Sympathetic Blockade

"I published the first medical case series on the use of the stellate ganglion block (SGB) for PTSD symptoms, and since then we've published ten studies, including clinical trials, and have performed over three thousand SGBs. The SGB is a medical procedure where an ultrasound-guided injection of a long-acting local anesthetic is performed in the side of the neck to temporarily "block" the nerve that controls the "fight or flight" response. This nerve (the cervical sympathetic chain) is a two-way conduit, where the parts

of the brain that control the fight or flight response (the central autonomic network) communicates with the body, and the body communicates back to those parts of the brain. We hypothesized that by temporarily blocking or "turning off" the two-way traffic between the body and those parts of the brain, the fight or flight response is allowed to reset, resulting in long-term relief of the associated anxiety symptoms. Over thirty peer-reviewed medical publications show that SGB is safe and results in significant long-term improvement in chronic anxiety symptoms associated with PTSD. The SGB involves only very minor discomfort and takes less than fifteen minutes to perform, with lasting benefits being seen in as little as thirty minutes."

—**Sean Mulvaney**, MD, former U.S. Navy SEAL
and U.S. Army physician

Stellate ganglion block (SGB) therapy, also known as cervical sympathetic blockade, is a medical procedure. As Sean Mulvaney describes above, it involves an injection of medicine, a local anesthetic, into the stellate ganglion, a bundle of nerves running through the neck belonging to the sympathetic nervous system. This is the division of our central nervous system that activates the "fight or flight" response, immediately arousing us to respond urgently to any form of danger or threat in our environment. This is an evolutionary mechanism that helped our ancestors survive the many dangers they faced—and it helps soldiers survive and react to the dangers they face. However, in people with PTSD and anxiety, this system is thought to be overactivated. Our understanding is that SGB works by turning down sympathetic nervous system activity, which results in less sympathetic arousal, inflammation, and pain sensitivity.

SGB is a brief outpatient procedure with virtually immediate relief for most people. Although the medicine typically wears off after several months, most people report that by the time it does, they have been sleeping and feeling much better—and many of the benefits remain. A bilateral SGB (both sides of the neck on two separate days) may enhance and extend the treatment benefits, and the treatment can be repeated every so often. Ketamine and SGB when used *in combination* are theorized to have synergistic effects, amplifying benefits. This procedure has been used in medicine for about one hundred years to treat certain types of headaches and is considered to be quite safe. This is often one of the first treatments I recommend to operators, because it is so effective and fast-acting, and because it treats PTSD, anxiety, anger, and insomnia.

Transcranial Magnetic Stimulation (TMS) or Magnetic e-Resonance Therapy (MeRT)

"Brain stimulation methods have demonstrated promise in mitigating Operator Syndrome symptoms by restoring disrupted neural communication. Magnetic EEG resonance therapy (MeRT), for instance, assesses an operator's brain activity, their alpha frequency, and applies individualized magnetic pulses at that frequency to impacted brain regions. As brain stimulation can modify neural activity over time, personalized therapies like MeRT offer unprecedented potential for addressing Operator Syndrome's lasting effects, even beyond deployments. Already adopted by special operations units, MeRT promotes overall health, performance, and career longevity, challenging the notion that care is necessary after someone becomes impaired."

—**Alexander J. Ring**, director of applied science at Wave Neuroscience

Transcranial magnetic stimulation (TMS) is a noninvasive, safe treatment for depression that uses magnetic coils to produce a series of pulses next to a patient's head. Though very mild, these magnetic pulses stimulate the activity of neurons in the brain region targeted. The strength and frequency of the pulses dictate how neuronal activity is altered (e.g., increasing or decreasing activity). TMS is typically administered five days a week for four to six weeks. Magnetic EEG resonance therapy (MeRT) is a variation of TMS that uses a sophisticated individualized alpha pulse frequency that is based on each patient's unique electroencephalogram (EEG) readings. The recent MeRT outcomes data collected from both active and inactive operators looks quite promising.[12] Anecdotally, I've also heard very satisfied reviews from a number of operators who have received this form of treatment.

Vestibular Therapy

Vestibular therapy is a form of physical therapy used to treat problems of the vestibular system, which is responsible for balance and spatial orientation. The goal is to improve the brain's ability to integrate and process sensory information from the vestibular system. This in turn will lead to improved balance and hand-eye coordination, reduced dizziness, and lower symptoms of nausea and fatigue. Imagine, for example, sitting in a special chair that tilts and rotates in order to move your inner ear in specific sequences to readjust particles in your inner ear.

Further Recommended Readings
- *Into the Ayahuasca: One Navy SEAL's Journey of Healing Through Plant Medicine* by Joe Schmuckatelli (2023)

---

12   Full disclosure: I serve as a scientific consultant to Wave Neuroscience.

CHAPTER 22

PERFORMANCE OPTIMIZATION

"If we reward rather than punish people for taking care of themselves, they'll be able to stay in the fight longer and perform at a higher level, benefiting the U.S. military just as much as the individual service member."

—**Kate Pate**, neurophysiology PhD

"The first SOF truth is 'humans are more important than hardware.' How many checks and services do you think our Special Operators get compared to a fighter jet or helicopter? Would the Air Force fly an F22 for five years without a regular scheduled maintenance cycle? Maintenance is the cornerstone of readiness. If we know the health effects of air pollution, toxins, repetitive trauma, sleep deprivation, blast overpressure, impact concussions, substance abuse, high op tempos, why are we not educating our operators? The first step in composite risk management (CRM) is: identify hazards. We clearly understand our weapons to be

life-sustaining equipment, yet we treated our bodies and minds as expendable items, like a rental car."

—**Geoff Dardia**, functional medicine certified health coach, U.S. Army Special Forces Master Sergeant, founder of SOF Health Initiative Program

"It's a mixed emotional response from the veteran SOF operators when we unravel their Operator Syndrome. First, there is intense gratitude that we've fixed their gut, optimized their nutrient status, treated their parasites, addressed heavy metals, balanced their hormones, improved their sleep, and got them off all or most medications. Then they get infuriated—pissed off that nobody did this sooner. They point out the careers, marriages, and even lives that could have been saved if this capability was more accessible."

—**Bryan Alexander Stepanenko**, MD, MPH, Institute for Functional Medicine certified practitioner, fellow of the American Academy of Family Physicians, U.S. Army Medical Corps, military functional medicine educator and practitioner

"To optimize Warfighter performance and reset operators after years of high tempo training and operations, a holistic, integrative approach is necessary. Optimization of hormones through good sleep practice, balanced exercise, and nutrition will provide the tools operators need to self-regulate. Approaches such as breathwork, yoga, acupuncture, HBOT, etc. are naturopathic and efficacious modalities that should be incorporated, depending on what resonates with the individual. There is not a one-size-fits-all

approach and it's important to realize that daily fluxes in physiology and metabolism will occur. Consistency is critical. Self-discipline is the purest form of self-love."

—**Karen R. Kelly**, PhD, physiologist at Warfighter Performance Naval Health Research Center

Operator Syndrome is a framework for understanding the many health effects and injuries that are inherent in a military career with special operations. This whole systems framework can also be used to guide efforts to minimize these injuries during a military career, to optimize performance, and to extend career longevity.

There are a variety of approaches to enhancing human performance, and many excellent multidisciplinary programs exist within the DOD. We still use concepts first developed and validated during World War II by the Office of Strategic Services Assessment Staff. These relate to mindset, as well as domains of physical, cognitive, and emotional functioning. Current human performance programs also incorporate medical and scientific advances in areas of diet, sleep, strength training, and recovery. One very simple formula for performance is as follows:

Training × Recovery = Performance

This is a good place to emphasize the importance of rest and recuperation. Recovery is half the equation that goes into performance. Too often we forget this or ignore it. Too often operators brush it off because it seems there is no time for it. But this is stinking thinking.

We know long and hard training is important for elite performance. Yet without adequate sleep, you are losing a lot of the desired benefits of your training. And it is not just sleep that we need for the recovery side of the performance equation. Diet matters too. So do positive social support and recovery practices that allow for quieting the mind and enhancing mindset. Any achievement of high performance must include approaches to maximize whole body and brain health—in other words, a whole systems approach.

I follow a basic outline in my coaching activities, but, of course, it must be adapted specifically for each individual—their past experiences, injuries, current situational realities, and goals. The lifestyle specifics (sleep, taming inflammation, diet, strength training, mindset) are covered in the next chapter and in other sections of this book. Also, though my coaching protocol is context-specific to operators, it can easily be adapted for any group. In my efforts with guys, I target seven broad categories.

Frueh's Operator Syndrome Coaching Protocol:

1. Understand your life history, current situation, and mission-specific goals.
2. Review Operator Syndrome domains as a framework. (I use the Operator Syndrome Survey as a tool to help structure the conversation.)
3. Address your lifestyle and habits: sleep, diet, fitness, recovery, personal relationships (marriages, children, etc.), occupational functioning.
4. Address your mindset.

5. Educate yourself on proactive medical testing, again using the syndrome framework. I encourage the following: cognitive functioning check, hormone levels check, sleep study, testing for heavy metals and parasites, neurological assessment, metabolic panels, psychiatric functioning check, etc.

6. Educate yourself on medical strategies to achieve, maintain, and improve health across the framework, as well as the ways to find these treatments (e.g., physical therapy, stellate ganglion block, ketamine, hormone therapies, MeRT, float tank, vestibular, speech pathology, psychiatric treatments, etc.).

7. Address your post-service career development and other life plans.

This was a short chapter, and it is light on specifics, but I hope the point is clear. The Operator Syndrome framework has practical value for every stage of an operator's life, from initial selection to mid-career to middle age, and beyond. The framework can be used to guide healing treatments and to optimize performance. This segues nicely into the next chapter, which provides information on the lifestyle and habits necessary for recovery and performance optimization.

Further Recommended Readings
- *Assessment of Men: Selection of Personnel for the Office of Strategic Services* by OSS Assessment Staff (Rinehart & Company, 1948)

CHAPTER 23

THE LIFESTYLE AND HABITS

"Everyone wants the easy button when it comes to Operator Syndrome. An injection, an ice bath, an all-meat diet. The reality is there's no easy solution. However, it can be very simple: Quit drinking alcohol. Prioritize your sleep. Learn how to down-regulate with breathing drills. Work out consistently. Eat like an athlete. You passed the hardest selection processes in the world—now use that same discipline and planning to take your life back. You were never meant to return to society to be average. Come back and demonstrate leadership in your life."
—Brent Phillips, former U.S. Marine Raider, CEO of SOFLETE

"When the grains of dark, rich, moist soil touch the hands while planting your first tomato plant of the season and a worm slithers between your fingers, surely the pond will provide this evening's meal. In the corner of your eye, you see a yellow blossom nearby and a honeybee enters to pollinate; the hives should be full again this season—it's all here. Everything needed to live a simple life. A homestead life. A cathartic, healing life of peace and tranquility

all at your fingertips allowing the past to fade and the future flourish. It's more than a lifestyle; it's truly living. I'm alive."

—**K.P.**, U.S. Air Force veteran, former intelligence operative, defense contractor

"I talk to my old teammates a lot. About normal stuff, how the kids are, what the weekend plans are going to be, and of course a little about work. I can be real with them about complex trauma. I can have fun with them about all the strange things we continue to grapple with."

—**Pete McGuyer**, U.S. Marine Chief Petty Officer, Reconnaissance and Marine Special Operations Command

Although professional interventions can really help mitigate the various conditions of Operator Syndrome, you must still put in hard work yourself. Effective and consistent lifestyle and habits are necessary. Obviously, the same is true for performance optimization.

Extensive training is required for elite performance in the military, and it is necessary for elite performance and good health in civilian life. You are training for a different mission once you are out of the military, but make no mistake—the mission sets will change, but they won't end. You may have fifty to eighty more years *after* your military service is over. Your families, communities, and nation continue to need you.

All of the following domains are critical: sleep, chronic inflammation, diet and gut health, recovery practices, exercise and movement, social support, mindset, and meaning and purpose in life. That's what this chapter is about. Let's dig in.

Sleep

You've probably figured out by now that I believe sleep is terribly important. So important, in fact, that for years I used a document I had written titled "The Operator's Sleep Manual."[13] I used it as an educational tool for the guys I coached. It pushed sleep forward as the single most important aspect of our lives to build healthy routines around. It also provided information on the bidirectional relationship between sleep and everything else in the syndrome (i.e., brain health, hormones, pain, depression, anger, and PTSD). The point was, if you do what it takes to sleep better, you will also have addressed the other elements of Operator Syndrome.

And who doesn't want to sleep better?

Getting good sleep is crucial for every aspect of our health and functioning. This means getting both sufficient quantity (seven to nine hours) and quality sleep (REM, slow-wave sleep) every night.

I won't belabor the points here again. Please refer to Chapter 3 for information on sleep and how to improve yours. Also, be aware that many of the treatments and lifestyle habits described in this book can help improve sleep indirectly. Treat your sympathetic nervous system arousal with stellate ganglion block therapy, and you are likely to relax and sleep better. Reduce chronic pain, and you will sleep better. And so on.

As your sleep improves, you will see benefits to your mood, cognition, energy, and overall health. Please make quality sleep a priority for the rest of your life.

Chronic Inflammation

Did you know that spending twenty minutes in a hot sauna three times a week can be a highly effective treatment for

---

13   This was essentially a very early draft of our Operator Syndrome medical paper.

depression? Randomized clinical trials have demonstrated this effect.

In 2019, my colleagues and I presented a scientific research review titled "The Role of Systemic Inflammation in Major Depressive Disorder and Implications for Novel Treatment Approaches" at the International Society for Affective Disorders annual conference.[14] To summarize: there is now strong medical evidence for an immune-mediated and causal component to depression.

Chronic inflammation also represents a causal mechanism in virtually *every* chronic illness of modern life: cancer, heart disease, pulmonary disease, autoimmune disorders, inflammatory bowel disease, obesity, and diabetes.

But let's back up. *What even is chronic, systemic inflammation?*

Think about a time when you cut your finger—maybe a paper cut or a minor kitchen mishap. After the bleeding stops, the wound turns red and swells up a little. It feels warm to the touch. This is an example of *acute* inflammation, our body's immune response to help prevent infection and heal the injury. Over the course of several days, as your finger mends, the visible inflammation recedes. Such inflammation is part of our immune system's complex physiological response to protect the body from pathogens and to support cellular health and tissue repair.

Inflammatory processes can also be *chronic* and *systemic*—involving inflammatory proteins that circulate through our bloodstream, affecting every cell in our body. When this occurs on a prolonged basis, we call it *chronic, systemic* inflammation. We can measure the severity of this type of inflammation in a number of ways, most commonly via blood tests that quantify

---

14   Christopher Frueh, et al, "The Role of Systemic Inflammation in Major Depressive Disorder and Implications for Novel Treatment Approaches," *Journal of Affective Disorders* 254 (2019): 139–140.

levels of various biomarkers, such as C-reactive protein (CRP), IFN-alpha, IL-6, and IL-10. All of these are correlated with chronic diseases—in fact, *all* of the chronic diseases.

Making matters worse, chronic diseases in turn contribute to inflammatory reactions, and therefore the relationship between disease and inflammation is bidirectional. In other words, a vicious cycle!

Our current understanding of mechanisms-of-action suggests that proinflammatory cytokines cross the blood-brain barrier and influence pathophysiologic domains. This includes decreased neurotrophic support, reduced brain monoamine levels, increased glutamate release and reuptake, increased oxidative stress, impaired brain plasticity, and activated neuroendocrine responses.

But why does this happen? And why is it so common?

The best explanation is that modern lifestyles in the industrialized world contribute to inflammation via behavioral habits (e.g., modern diets, sedentary lives, poor sleep routines) and environmental exposures that are incompatible with our evolutionary history as a species. Among other things, this includes a highly plausible theory that modernity has led to a loss of natural exposure to previously available sources of anti-inflammatory, immunoregulatory signaling (i.e., "germs" or "old friends") that were previously common in our soil, food, and gut microbiota. (If you want to nerd out, look up "tolerogenic microorganisms" and the "pathogen host defense" theory).

Anti-Inflammatory Habits to Optimize Performance, Wellness, and Longevity

"Cold exposure was part of the human evolutionary experience for hundreds of thousands of years before the modern age. The cold that many special operators or expeditionary forces experience is usually

considered part of their hardships, but ironically it may also help protect them from extraordinary stressors. The ones I've worked with in cold water immersion tell me the cold helps reset their nervous system and restores their sense of calm and well-being."

—**Thomas P Seager**, PhD, Associate Professor, Engineering Business Practices, Arizona State University

The good news is you almost certainly don't need medications to help manage chronic systemic inflammation.[15] Lifestyle modifications and certain regular habits can massively reduce it. These include the following:

- **Exercise.** A sedentary lifestyle induces systemic inflammation. Conversely, exercise has a powerful anti-inflammatory affect.
- **Sleep.** Sleep dysregulation—insomnia, jet lag, shift work, sleep deprivation—contributes to systemic inflammation. Make sure your sleep hygiene is dialed in. This means scheduling sufficient time in bed, going to bed at the same time every night, and sleeping in a dark, silent, and cool bedroom.
- **Timing the circadian clock.** Epidemiological data show that 80 percent of the general population is living a "shift-work lifestyle" (e.g., chronic circadian rhythm disruption) and may be at risk for chronic diseases associated with inflammation. Deploying strategies that optimize the circadian lifestyle, timing of therapies, and targeting specific circadian elements may be highly beneficial. Going to bed at the same

---

15   Portions of this chapter were previously adapted for and published in *Men's Journal* Everyday Warrior series in 2023.

time every night and getting five to ten minutes of early morning direct sunlight on your eyes can work wonders.

- **Time-restricted feeding (TRF) or intermittent fasting.** Restricting eating to within a narrow window of time (twelve or eight hours, or even less) every day may offer a range of health benefits associated with reduced inflammation, including weight management and improved mood and cognition. In research conducted with mice, TRF (using a ten-hour feeding window) prevents obesity and metabolic syndrome even when the mice are allowed to eat the same number of calories that caused other non-TRF mice to rapidly gain weight. A TRF approach in humans may have a similar benefit and may also enhance cellular defenses against metabolic stress. It is also probably more consistent with the feeding pattern of our ancestors.

- **Diet.** Eating a whole foods diet (e.g., a Mediterranean or ketogenic diet) that minimizes added sugar, processed foods, alcohol, and refined grains—and maximizes healthy fats, quality proteins, fiber, natural vegetables, and some fruit—has an anti-inflammatory effect. Following the Mediterranean diet or a diet low on foods from the Dietary Inflammatory Index is associated with a lower risk of depression and inflammation. Eating highly processed junk food increases both. Small changes can make a difference. For example, flavonoid-rich dark chocolate (two grams with 70 percent cocoa) reduces DNA damage, improves the nucleus integrity of cells, improves biochemical parameters (total cholesterol, triglycerides, and LDL cholesterol), and reduces waist circumference. An anti-inflammatory diet is associated with reduced all-cause mortality. Eat wisely and live better for longer.

- **Hydration.** Drink plenty of water, about eighty to 120 ounces a day—more, if you are sweating heavily.
- **Supplementation.** Certain naturally occurring compounds within foods and dietary supplements help reduce inflammation. This includes curcumin-rich turmeric, vitamin D, and omega-3 fatty acids. Other supplements help promote cellular health, including NAD+, NMN, and B vitamins.
- **Pre- and probiotics.** As we learn more about the connection between gut microbiota and systemic inflammation, evidence suggests probiotic supplementation, as well as foods that support gut health (e.g., fermented foods, bone broth), are anti-inflammatory. Fermented foods include yogurt, kefir, miso, and anything that is naturally pickled without the use of vinegar.
- **Stress management.** Psychological stress leads to increased production of pro-inflammatory cytokines. Activities that help manage levels of perceived stress and responses to stress have an anti-inflammatory effect. Recovery practices have shown profound benefits. Examples include meditation, yoga, stretching, jiujitsu, religious or spiritual practices, unplugging from digital connections, spending time outdoors (e.g., "forest bathing"), soothing hobbies, and positive social support.
- **Sauna bathing, cold immersion, float therapy.** Hyperthermia (e.g., Finnish-style sauna bathing) is associated with reduced systemic inflammation and a range of health benefits, including reduced risk of

vascular and cardiovascular diseases, neurocognitive diseases, pulmonary diseases, and all-cause mortality. Other recovery practices—cold immersion (ice baths), float tank therapy—also appear to have powerful anti-inflammatory benefits.

Chronic, systemic inflammation plays a powerful role in the etiology of virtually all chronic diseases. It is primarily caused by our modern lifestyle and dietary habits. Modifying your habits to live a more "ancient" lifestyle will reduce inflammation, enhance metabolic and immune functioning, and improve your overall health and functioning.

Diet and Gut Health

There is a tight connection between our gut health and brain functioning, metabolic health, psychological health, performance, and overall wellness. Recent research shows that the gut microbiome, made up of bacteria, fungi, protozoa, and viruses, plays an essential role in the central nervous system via its effects on digestion, immune functioning, systemic inflammation, the hypothalamic-pituitary axis, and many other aspects of health.

The vast majority of the research on the microbiome has been conducted with animals (typically mice), but we now have a few small studies with human subjects. An unhealthy gut microbiome is associated with depression and anxiety. Our gut microbiota interacts with the reward system of the brain as it relates to our use of food and drugs and our pursuit of pleasure.

In 2020, my colleague Alok Madan (a coauthor on the Operator Syndrome medical paper) led a study[16] with

---

16 Alok Madan, et al, "The Gut Microbiota Is Associated with Psychiatric Symptom Severity and Treatment Outcome among Individuals with Serious Mental Illness," *Journal of Affective Disorders* 264 (2020): 98–106.

hospitalized psychiatric patients to examine the gut microbiomes of people with severe mental illnesses. Patients reported their clinical symptoms through a battery of self-report questionnaires related to psychiatric symptoms and functioning, and then provided fecal samples shortly after hospital admission. We worked with a team of microbiologists to sequence the DNA of the bacteria and identify different types of bacteria.

We were able to retroactively identify patients at the start of treatment who did not benefit from their care, based solely on a fecal sample! Much more research is needed before we can fully understand the gut and its role in health in behavior, its multiple roles within our body, and how best to care for it—but we know it is vital for our well-being.

The Microbiome

Our gut microbiome weighs up to five pounds and has two hundred times the number of genes found in the human genome. It is symbiotic—not parasitic—to us. We *need* our gut microbes, and they need us. We survive and thrive together, and therefore we must take good care of it. A healthy gut is an essential component of health, performance, and general wellness. So, how do we best take care of this mysterious universe of organisms that live within us? The following are lifestyle habits that promote gut health:

1. Eat a healthy diet with plenty of fiber, lean protein, fats, and water.
2. Include prebiotics in your diet, plant fibers that facilitate growth of healthy bacteria, such as apples, bananas, barley, berries, cocoa, flaxseed, garlic, oats, onions, tomatoes, soybeans, and wheat.

3. Include probiotics in your diet, such as yoghurt, kefir, vinegar with active cultures, fermented pickles and sauerkraut, kimchi, etc. You can also take dietary probiotic supplements.

4. Eliminate or minimize consumption of processed food, junk food, fast food, soda, and added sugar.

5. Consider intermittent fasting or a time-restricted feeding approach.

6. Consider whether you have food sensitivities or allergies that might benefit from a special diet (e.g., a low-FODMAP diet, which is especially helpful for chronic symptoms of irritable bowel syndrome).

7. Exercise on a regular basis—especially strength training.

8. Pursue high-quality sleep, and plenty of it.

9. Eliminate or minimize alcohol use.

10. Regularly engage in meditation, yoga, stretching, prayer, or other recovery practices.

11. Consider past exposures to toxic chemicals, heavy metals, excessive smoke, etc., that may require medical consultation.

12. Spend time outdoors.

Our scientific understanding of the gut microbiota is still at a very early stage, and it is true that most human studies to date only examine the strength of the *association* between psychological functioning and gut health. From Psychology 101 we are reminded that "correlation is not causation." Nevertheless, with what we know now and what we hypothesize from that knowledge, there is every reason to take good care of your gut health—and absolutely no reason not to.

The best part is that whatever is good for your gut is also good for your weight, heart, lungs, muscles, skeletal system, skin, brain, cognitive functioning, wellness, and functional performance—and I mean performance in literally every important area of personal and professional life.

As an example, consider my own personal dietary protocol. I take a daily intermittent fasting approach, with a feeding window of about six to nine hours most days. My first meal of the day is a smoothie made with a varied mixture of frozen fruit (e.g., blueberries, raspberries, blackberries, strawberries, cherries, pineapple), fresh fruits (bananas, apples, exotics), vegetables (carrots, spinach), dairy (yoghurt, kefir), avocado, MCT or olive oil, and a blend of nuts (walnuts, pecans), seeds (flax, chia, hemp, pumpkin, sesame, sunflower), cacao nibs, a variety of so-called "superfood" powders (e.g., ginger, beetroot, cinnamon, mushroom extracts, noni, maca, acai), shredded coconut, a half cup of oatmeal, and unsweetened protein powder.

I prep a week's worth of a dry blend of nuts, seeds, powders, and oatmeal every weekend using two-cup plastic containers. This allows me to blend and eat my first meal of the day in about fifteen minutes. My preference for protein powders is unsweetened casein powder, collagen powder (with multiple peptides), and grass-fed beef isolate and egg white powder.

For dinner, I usually eat beef or seafood with a salad or a large serving of mixed vegetables (baked, stewed, or stir-fried). Cottage cheese, mixed nuts, and hard-boiled eggs make for easy protein snacks during the day.

If you're wondering where I stand on carbs, I do eat them, but in moderation. Typically, I have a half-cup of oatmeal in my first meal and one to two pieces of bread at my second meal. I bake my own bread using my homemade sourdough starter (which is so much easier than we have all been led to believe) and organically grown whole-grain ancient and heirloom wheats that have been stone-milled. As a result, my homemade bread has lots of healthy fiber, nutrients, and fermented dough (which is filled with lactobacilli, a healthy bacteria)—and no unhealthy ingredients or cheap oils.

If my dietary protocol sounds a little difficult or too time-consuming, it's actually not. It is easy once you've put in a few reps, and it becomes extremely time-efficient. If it sounds too earthy, nutty, or crunchy for you, all I can say is this: Try it for two weeks. You are likely to feel so much better that you never return to your old dietary habits. You don't have to be perfect—I'm certainly not—and even small changes can be transformative. *Bon appétit*!

Recovery Practices

We all need time to unplug, quiet our mind, encourage our imagination, and renew our connection with the universe. I refer to activities that help us do this as "recovery practices." There are lots of them, plenty of options, and you should use several of them—every day, every week, every month, and every year.

These are not frivolous or woo-woo activities. They can provide incredible benefits, including reduced inflammation, better sleep, heightened concentration, and soothed rage. They also might just bring some peace of mind. They matter to our souls.

Most of the practices listed below are solitary activities, which I believe are important. Blaise Pascal (1623–1662) wrote, "All of humanity's problems stem from man's inability to sit quietly in a room alone." Stillness is even recommended in the Bible. Psalm 46:10 directs us to "be still and know that I am God."

Here are some of the recovery practices that many operators and spouses have used and found to be extremely helpful:

- Hot sauna
- Cold immersion
- Float tank therapy
- Jiujitsu, tai chi
- Time with animals—dogs, cats, horses, etc.
- Time in nature, sunlight, "forest bathing"
- Yoga, stretching
- Meditation
- Prayer
- Hobbies
- Gardening
- Music (performing or listening)
- Handcrafts (wood, leather, metals)
- Journaling
- Arts and creativity (drawing, painting, writing poetry or books)
- Cooking
- Reading, learning

Exercise and Movement

All of you tactical athletes, please don't skip through this section. There may be some surprises—including how to do strength training without further damage to your joints.

You've probably lifted weights your entire life. However, after a career in special operations, your mission set changes and, therefore, so should your training. You train for the mission, right? Well, after your military service is over, you no longer need to be prepared to ruck with 120 pounds of kit and gear—nor should you.

Much of the chronic pain that operators experience is from the constant "wear and tear" on joints and spine. Running and lifting heavy with free weights are especially hard on the joints, and they are no longer as necessary as they once were. Time to switch things up, because you will need your knees, back, and shoulders for decades more to come.

Your new long-term goals should be to maintain health, strength, and functionality. You want to be mobile and independent, able to stand up out of a chair, pick up your grandchildren, and enjoy many other activities of daily life until the day you die. Sarcopenia is a special enemy that you must defend against for the long haul.

Sarcopenia is the gradual loss of skeletal muscle mass, strength, and functioning. It typically begins at some point in our thirties. People who are physically inactive can lose 3 to 5 percent of their muscle mass each decade; even active people are likely to have some muscle loss. Any loss of muscle is a concern, because it lessens strength and mobility.

The pace of muscle loss accelerates around age seventy-five. Sarcopenia in elderly people is a major cause of frailty and increases the likelihood of falls and bone fractures. Primary causes of muscle loss are declines in hormones, systemic inflammation, less physical activity, changes in cellular health, and malnutrition (e.g., inadequate protein intake). The good news is that sarcopenia can be prevented or reversed with dietary changes and strength training.

Skeletal muscle is the largest organ in the human body. It is essential for physical functioning, optimal hormonal balance, cardiac health, bone density, pulmonary health, and metabolic functioning. According to a 2020 scientific literature review,[17] strength training in combination with a healthy diet (e.g., sufficient protein intake) is the most effective way to prevent or slow the progression of sarcopenia.

Strength training involves lifting, pushing, or pulling movements in order to load and overload the muscle so that it will adapt by getting stronger. All major muscle groups should be targeted with heavy resistance, or heavy loads, two or three times a week, with at least one rest day between working out the same muscle group. At the end of this section, I will share my strength training protocol with variable resistance bands. It might surprise you, but it is very effective and also gentle on the joints—so much so that my decades of joint and chronic lower back pain have disappeared.

Dietary and Supplementation Recommendations

Strength training by itself is wasted effort. A healthy diet is the other essential component to staving off sarcopenia. An evidence-based nutritional support approach synergizes with strength training.

Protein is critical for a diet that supports the development of skeletal muscle. The first thing you need to know is that the U.S. recommended daily allowance (RDA) for protein intake has been unchanged for decades—and is woefully inadequate for strength training. The second thing you need to know is that total daily protein intake is the most important dietary contribution to muscle mass. Older adults typically consume insufficient amounts of protein. So how much protein do adults really need to provide maximum stimulation of muscle

---

17   James McKendry, et al, "Nutritional Supplements to Support Resistance Exercise in Countering the Sarcopenia of Aging," *Nutrients* 12, no. 7 (2020): 2057.

protein synthesis (MPS)? And what are the best forms of protein to consume?

1. Adults require 1.2 grams of protein for every kilogram of body weight (one kilogram equals 2.205 pounds) daily to provide maximum MPS. For example, a two-hundred-pound person needs 90.7 grams of protein every day. Some scientists think even this is too low, recommending one gram of protein for every pound of body weight. I subscribe to this perspective. There is also evidence that we need even more protein as we get older.

2. The National Health and Nutrition Examination Survey (2007–2016) found a strong association between daily protein intake and disability. People who consumed more than one gram of protein per kilogram of weight each day had 22 percent decreased odds for functional disability. The European Society for Clinical Nutrition and Metabolism have recently recommended that older adults should consume between one and 1.5 grams of protein per kilogram of weight each day. High-protein intake equals less disability.

3. Not all proteins are created equal. They can be objectively scored for their quality using the protein digestibility-corrected amino acid score (PDCAAS) or the digestible indispensable amino acid score (DIAAS). Results of these analyses show that animal-derived proteins are superior to soy, pea, and most other plant-based proteins.

4. Protein distribution throughout the day is also important and contributes significant benefits to MPS. This means it's important to consume twenty-five to

fifty grams of protein at every meal throughout the day, possibly with smaller protein snacks in between meals.

5. Contrary to popular belief, a higher protein intake is not detrimental to kidney or bone health. In fact, a higher protein intake is probably beneficial to bone density health and may help reduce risk of hip and other bone fractures common among older adults.

Creatine is found in meat and fish, and its primary function is to facilitate the transmission of high-energy phosphates in the production of adenosine triphosphate (ATP). Start by taking five grams of creatine monohydrate four times a day for one week, followed by an ongoing maintenance dose of five grams a day. Creatine is safe, well-tolerated, and an important component of building and maintaining skeletal muscle. If you do strength training, you should supplement with creatine.

Other dietary supplements can include the following:

1. Vitamin D3 plus K can be used to combat deficiencies in vitamin D, which are common in most Americans and associated with musculoskeletal disease.
2. Leucine, an essential amino acid, is beneficial if overall protein intake is insufficient. This may be especially important for people who eat plant-based proteins as their primary source of protein (e.g., vegetarians).
3. Omega-3 polyunsaturated fatty acids (n3-PUFA) are commonly found in fish oil and may be especially important during periods of relative inactivity (e.g., during illness or recovery periods).

To provide a specific example of useful strength training, I will share my own protocol. I'm no tactical athlete, but I do okay in a T-shirt. In 2020, I completed the "Murph Challenge" in seventy-two minutes—not a SEAL-trained time, but not bad for a fifty-six-year-old nerd with a PhD.[18] However, it took a good week before my elbows would cooperate again. After that (along with the discovery of a chronic medical illness), I decided to completely change up my strength training protocol.

Now I use a variable-resistance band system[19] that involves working out with large, flat circular bands, a shoulder-width Olympic bar with hooks for the bands, and a plate to thread the band under, which prevents ankle rolls. This system fits easily in my carry-on luggage when I travel. At home, I use a vibration plate, but when I'm on the road, I use a simple plate.

Variable-resistance bands work with your strength curve instead of against it as free weights do. What this means is that at the start of the motion, when you are at your weakest and before the band has been stretched, the resistance is at its lightest. As you proceed through the motion, the band stretches and the resistance increases gradually, matching your strength curve. This means that acute and repetitive stress injuries are far less likely to occur. Over time, the injuries you do have may heal, and your chronic joint pain is likely to fade.

Using bands instead of free weights also means you can go to failure and beyond (i.e., partial reps). For this reason, I only do *one set* per muscle group. To get the most out of that one set, you really have to make full effort. This means doing as many reps (i.e., fifteen to forty) as you possibly can, and then

---

18 The "Murph Challenge," a fundraiser for the Lieutenant Michael P. Murphy Memorial Scholarship, involves two miles of running, one hundred pull-ups, two hundred sit-ups, and three hundred squats, all while wearing a twenty-pound vest.

19 I use the Jaquish Biomedical X3 variable-resistance band system developed by Dr. John Jaquish.

continuing to do partial reps until you are no longer able to move the bar more than an inch.

On "push days," I do four sets, one each of the following: chest press, triceps extension, shoulder press, and squats. On "pull days" I do four sets of the following: dead lift, calf raise, bent-over row, and bicep curl. This targets all major muscle groups. I hit these four to six days a week, and each workout is less than fifteen minutes.

I've been using this approach for two years now with good results—and 95 percent of the chronic joint and back pain I lived with for decades has disappeared. I get that you still want to look dangerous beyond your military career, and with this training method, you will continue to.

Social Support

In Chapter 15, I reminded you that "no man is an island." We evolved from hunter-gatherer tribes that were highly dependent on each other for individual and collective survival. This means that humans as a species evolved to thrive on positive connections with other humans. We suffer profoundly when we do not have these connections. Throughout our evolutionary history, it has literally been in our DNA to be social creatures.

Loneliness kills us.

Many operators feel the loss of their tribe after they leave the military. You can't replace the "Brotherhood," but you can make new friends and find respect among colleagues and coworkers in civilian life. You will have new neighbors, a new job, and you will attend new churches and schools. Your family will, too, and you'll find a few connections using their social network.

Do not sit around alone. Go make friends and do stuff with them.

Mindset

The way we think about ourselves and the world around us has a powerful impact on everything. This includes our emotions, behaviors, physiological state, our sense of purpose and meaning, and our relationships. A productive cognitive mindset involves being optimistic, resilient, compassionate, mindful, and keeping a clear line of sight on your purpose and mission in life. But it isn't easy to maintain this mindset, especially when you are suffering from depression, anxiety, anger, fatigue, grief, or disillusionment. So, what can you do?

Consider some of the following issues that can take you off track:

- Fear of failure, embarrassment, rejection
- Negativity about other people
- Self-destructive habits, like drinking too much
- Guilt or shame
- Memories of past failures or traumas

How can you be more aware of these cognitive disrupters? Consider doing the following:

- Take inventory. Have honest conversations with yourself and others you trust.
- Get evaluated by a professional of whatever stripe that makes sense for you.
- Train with an expert, such as a coach or therapist.

What can you do to stay on course with your cognitive mindset? Here are some examples to follow:

- Try recovery practices, such as meditation, prayer, breath work, or float therapy.
- Prioritize family time.
- Engage in hobbies and relaxation habits.
- Strive to be curious and humble.
- Seek out regular emotional intimacy with people you care for.
- Give regular attention to your purpose.

It may not sound like much, but if we tune into our inner dialogue on a consistent basis, we become more aware of and more constructive with our mindset. That can make a huge positive difference in our lives. It can be the difference between despair and hope.

"Helping SOF orient toward a process- and value-oriented life, as opposed to an outcome-oriented one, may be all the difference they need. Consider the U.S. withdrawal from Afghanistan. An outcome-oriented SO would likely see only loss and failure. A process-oriented SO is more likely to appreciate all their experiences gained, lessons learned, relationships built, and lives saved."
—**Michael Vollmer**, PsyD, U.S. Navy Lieutenant, Military Sealift Command and SEAL, licensed clinical psychologist

Meaning and Purpose

For well over a millennium, philosophers and theologians have advised us of the colossal importance of meaning and purpose. In more recent decades, a strong body of social science research has shown that having a strong sense of meaning and purpose in life is linked with better health and living longer. (It is also associated with earning more money.)

It's difficult to leave a career and community behind, especially when that career was so critically important, dangerous, and exhilarating. You were a highly elite performer, working closely with other elite performers, and you had all the cool toys. Many operators feel adrift after military discharge or retirement. It's natural to wonder if your productive days are behind you. But they don't have to be—nor should they be.

You voluntarily served your nation, accepting the possibility of mortal danger every day. You have a servant's heart. It is within you to continue to serve. You have rare skills and unique personal qualities. Your family, community, and nation continue to need you.

Further Recommended Readings

- *Food: What the Heck Should I Eat?* by Mark Hyman, MD (Little, Brown Spark, 2018)
- *Metabolical: The Lure and Lies of Processed Food, Nutrition, and Modern Medicine* by Robert H. Lustig, MD, MSL (Harper Wave, 2021)
- *A Silent Fire: The Story of Inflammation, Diet, and Disease* by Shilpa Ravella (W.W. Norton, 2022)
- *Outlive: The Science & Art of Longevity* by Peter Attia, MD (Harmony Books, 2023)
- *Forever Strong: A New, Science-Based Strategy for Aging Well* by Dr. Gabrielle Lyon (Atria Books, 2023)

CHAPTER 24

CHARLIE MIKE

"I knew when I joined the special operations community that it was a huge possibility and that I could wind up severely physically injured or dead, because the nature of the job and because it was during a time of war. I accepted that risk. What I did not expect were the invisible injuries that seemed to appear out of nowhere not too long after I retired. I still deal with the repercussions of the job, but I have come leaps and bounds from where I was three years ago, because of the people that I have in my life, the work I have put into making myself better, and my faith."

—**Eddie Gallagher**, former U.S. Navy SEAL, coauthor of *The Man in the Arena: From Fighting ISIS to Fighting for My Freedom*

"You must always remember that it was you who chose the hard path. It was never meant to be easy, but the hard was also never meant to apply to the physical alone. It would always be difficult physically, psychologically, emotionally, and existentially. Now comes the time when, just as you took responsibility for handling the physical challenges, you need to take responsibility for the other

challenges as well. No one is coming to save you, but there are a great many coaches, psychologists, chaplains, etc., who can teach you the skills to get to the next level."

—**Dr. Preston B. Cline**, director of research and education at the Mission Critical Team Institute

Operator Syndrome is not an identity. Don't ever let it become one. It is a framework to help you better understand and guide your health and functioning. It is a whole systems perspective toward understanding the interconnected pattern of medical, psychological, and social injuries that are common to operators.

Allostatic load refers to the accumulated burden of physiological, neurological, and neuroendocrine weight. This is an abstract term, because much of that "load" is not easy to quantify or measure. Derived from a military career in special operations, your accumulated allostatic load has been extraordinarily high. Injuries are inevitable. But there can absolutely be tremendous, game-changing healing and recovery ahead.

This recovery will require you to be persistent in the face of many obstacles. Some of these obstacles will be familiar to you, while others will not. You must continue to educate yourself. Be patient with the trial-and-error process of finding which of the many different treatments out there will be the right ones for you.

There will be dark periods when it seems you are back at square one. Setbacks are inevitable. Just when you think you are doing well, stuff can happen—plan in advance for this. Develop a safety plan. Write out an SOP for how you will respond when you do—predictably and once more—feel discouraged, frustrated, sick, or in despair.

Going forward, honor your family and friends. Remain connected to the "Brotherhood." Chase your purpose. Continue to serve others.

Focus carefully on your sleep, diet, exercise, social relationships, mindset, and meaning in life. You know the drill.

Approach your professional treatments with patience and determination. Stay on top of all appointments and follow-up exams. Make adjustments as necessary. Also, don't forget the basics of healthcare: regular primary and dental care appointments.

————

This book is dedicated to Claude E. Brocklebank and Mrs. John R. Beane, who, in 1898, retrieved my great-grandfather from Camp Wikoff and nursed him back to health in her home. I can only hope that I have helped satisfy the debt for what she paid forward.

————

In closing, for all the operators, I'll remind you once more: You served for beautiful reasons—for your comrades, your family, and your country. Your service carried the will and authority of a democratic nation behind it. Perhaps the best advice I can give every operator is to approach your health like you did your career in special operations. Never quit, never get out of the fight, find a way around or through, get off the X, solve for X, check on your teammates, continue mission.

"…either by chance or destiny—stepped up and led, and together, from what they accomplished, became immortal."

—**Hawk Slater**, U.S. Navy SEAL (Ret.),
Philadelphia firefighter, from his speech given to the
Penn State University football team in 2012

ABOUT THE AUTHOR

Chris Frueh, PhD, is a clinical psychologist and Professor of Psychology at the University of Hawaii, Hilo. He has over thirty years of professional experience working with military veterans, service members, special operators, and private defense contractors. He has conducted clinical trials, epidemiology, historical epidemiology, and neuroscience research. He has coauthored over three hundred scientific publications, including a graduate textbook on adult psychopathology. Previously, he was a tenured professor at the Medical University of South Carolina and Baylor College of Medicine.

He has testified before U.S. Congress and served as a paid consultant for the Department of Defense, Veterans Affairs, the U.S. State Department, and the National Board of Medical Examiners. He has also published commentaries in *National Review*, *Huffington Post*, *The New York Times*, *Time*, *Men's Journal*, and *Special Operations Association of America*. He has been quoted or cited in *The Wall Street Journal*, *The Economist*, *The Washington Post*, *Scientific American*, *Stars and Stripes*, *USA Today*, *Men's Health*, *Los Angeles Times*, *Reuters*, *Associated Press*, and *NBC News*, among others.

He devotes time to SEAL Future Foundation, Special Operations Association of America, Boulder Crest Foundation, Military Special Operations Family Collaborative, The Mission Within, VETS, Inc., and Big Country Veterans. He has also published nine historical crime novels, including *They Die Alone* (2013) and, most recently, *A Season Past* (2019).